Care Bundles in Emergency Medicine

TIMOTHY WILLIAMSON
MB ChB, BSc (Hons)
NIHR Academic Clinical Fellow in Medical Education
University of Leicester, UK

Acute Care Common Stem Trainee (Emergency Medicine)
University Hospitals of Leicester, UK

BILAL SALMAN
MB ChB, BSc (Hons)
ST3 Acute Care Common Stem Trainee (Emergency Medicine)
West Midlands Deanery, UK

RACHAEL BODDY
MB ChB, MRCP, FCEM
Consultant in Emergency Medicine
Heart of England NHS Foundation Trust
Birmingham, UK

MATTHEW COOKE
MB ChB, FCEM, FRCS(Ed), DipIMC, MF MLM
Professor of Emergency Medicine
University of Warwick, UK

Consultant in Emergency Medicine
Heart of England NHS Foundation Trust
Birmingham, UK

Foreword by
PROFESSOR PETER CAMERON
Immediate Past President, International Federation for Emergency Medicine
Chair, Emergency Medicine, HMC Doha, Qatar
Academic Director, Emergency and Trauma Centre
The Alfred Hospital, Monash University
Melbourne, Australia

Radcliffe Publishing
London • New York

Radcliffe Publishing Ltd
St Mark's House
Shepherdess Walk
London N1 7BQ
United Kingdom

www.radcliffehealth.com

British Library Cataloguing in Publication Data

A catalogue record for this book is available from the British Library.

ISBN-13: 978 184619 442 9

The paper used for the text pages of this book is FSC® certified. FSC (The Forest Stewardship Council®) is an international network to promote responsible management of the world's forests.

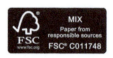

Typeset by Darkriver Design, Auckland, New Zealand
Manufacturing managed by 21six

Contents

Foreword

It is a great pleasure to write the Foreword to this innovative publication from some of the leaders in evidence-based emergency care in the UK. The very nature of emergency medical practice requires fast decision-making in a highly pressured environment. Making this simple, by identifying the components of emergency care that *must* be done, is very important. Ensuring that the best evidence available is used to back the recommendations is equally important. For all the complexity of current practice in emergency care, most of the management interventions that have good evidence and which make a difference to outcome are actually very straightforward. Getting all this information together into one small tome is useful both for the clinician practising in the field and for managers trying to assess whether quality care is being delivered. I would envisage that some health services may use the content of this book to identify key processes to audit for quality care. I congratulate the authors on this timely addition to the emergency literature.

Professor Peter Cameron
Immediate Past President, International Federation
for Emergency Medicine
Chair, Emergency Medicine, HMC Doha, Qatar
Academic Director, Emergency and Trauma Centre
The Alfred Hospital, Monash University
Melbourne, Australia
August 2014

Preface

What is a care bundle?

A care bundle is defined as a group of specific but non-prescriptive, evidence-based components that, when performed collectively and reliably, have been proven to improve patient outcomes. This book employs this care bundle approach as propagated by the Institute for Healthcare Improvement. Each care bundle component should satisfy the following criteria:

- ➲ each component must be **based on sound evidence**
- ➲ delivery of each component must be **in need of improvement**
- ➲ delivery of each component must be **achievable in terms of resources**
- ➲ no component should be a **major source of controversy**
- ➲ the delivery of each component must be **measurable**.

Why this book?

Emergency medicine care bundles aim to support those in emergency care to provide focused management plans for common presentations encountered in the emergency department by trainees and consultants.

Care bundles are focused on the initial intervention and are specific to the initial resuscitation and management that often precedes specialist treatment. This enables a clearer response from the emergency care team, whose aim is to make a difference to the patient's long-term outcome from the first few steps of treatment in the emergency department.

TW, BS, RB, MC
August 2014

Abbreviations

AST	aspartate transaminase
bd	twice daily
BHCG	beta human chorionic gonadotrophin
BNP	brain natriuretic peptide
BP	blood pressure
Ca^{2+}	calcium
CK	creatine kinase
COPD	chronic obstructive pulmonary disease
CRP	C-reactive protein
CRT	capillary refill time
C-Spine	cervical spine
CT	computed tomography
CTKUB	CT kidneys, ureter, bladder
CTPA	CT pulmonary angiography
CVP	central venous pressure
DVT	deep vein thrombosis
ECG	electrocardiogram
ESR	erythrocyte sedimentation rate
FBC	full blood count
GCS	Glasgow Coma Scale
GP	general practitioner
GTN	glyceryl trinitrate
HONK	hyperosmolar hyperglycaemic non-ketotic coma
HR	heart rate
IM	intramuscular
INR	international normalised ratio
IO	intraosseous
ITU	intensive therapy unit/intensive treatment unit
IV	intravenous
K^+	potassium
KUB	kidneys, ureter and bladder
LDH	lactate dehydrogenase

LFT	liver function tests
MC&S	microscopy, culture and sensitivity
MRI	magnetic resonance imaging
NBM	nil by mouth
NEXUS	National Emergency X-Radiography Utilization Study
NG	nasogastric
NSTEMI	non-ST elevation myocardial infarction
PCI	purcutaneous coronary intervention
PE	pulmonary embolus
PEFR	peak expiratory flow rate
PICU	paediatric intensive care unit
PO	per oral
prn	as required
qds	four times a day
RR	respiratory rate
SC	subcutaneous
STAT	immediately
STEMI	ST elevation myocardial infarction
tds	three times a day
TFT	thyroid function test
TIA	transient ischaemic attack
U&E	urea and electrolytes
USS	ultrasound scan
UTI	urinary tract infection

THE UNIVERSAL CARE BUNDLE

There are certain aspects of care that are universal to all patients. This care bundle should be reviewed before discharge, transfer or handover of all patients.

- ➲ Does the patient know and understand his or her diagnosis?
- ➲ Has a plan been explained to the patient?
- ➲ Does the patient understand his or her medication and its possible adverse effects?
- ➲ Does the patient know when to seek help?
- ➲ Have the symptoms been controlled?
- ➲ Has appropriate information been passed on to the clinicians and carers?

1

TRAUMA

For trauma cases it is presumed that appropriate resuscitation will be under-taken according to Advanced Trauma Life Support guidelines when required. Each care bundle therefore applies to the specific injury.

> *Advanced Trauma Life Support.* 8th ed. Chicago, IL: American College of Surgeons; 2008.

Head injury (GCS score <15)[1]

1. Record Glasgow Coma Scale (GCS) score
2. Always consider cervical spine (C-spine) injury
3. Record pupil size and response
4. Imaging: consider need for computed tomography (CT) of the head
5. Full evaluation of any wounds to the head
6. Obtain early senior and/or intensive treatment unit (ITU), anaesthetic or neurosurgical opinion as required

Additional information

Glasgow Coma Scale (minimum score 3, maximum score 15)

Best motor response		Best verbal response		Eyes open	
Obeys commands	6	Orientated	5	Spontaneously	4
Localises pain	5	Confused	4	Verbal command	3
Withdraws from pain	4	Inappropriate words	3	Pain	2
Abnormal flexion	3	Incomprehensible sounds	2	No response	1
Abnormal extension	2	No vocalisations	1		
No movement	1				

Selecting patients for CT imaging of the head

Criteria for immediate request for CT scan of the head (adults)

- ➲ GCS score <13 on initial assessment in the emergency department
- ➲ GCS score <15 at 2 hours post injury on assessment in the emergency department
- ➲ Vomiting more than once
- ➲ Post-traumatic seizure
- ➲ Suspected open or depressed skull fracture
- ➲ Focal neurological deficit
- ➲ Any signs of basal skull fracture (haemotympanum, 'panda' eyes, cerebrospinal fluid leakage from the ear or nose, Battle's sign)
- ➲ Amnesia >30 minutes prior to injury

Immediate request for CT scan of the head, provided patient has experienced some loss of consciousness or amnesia since the injury (adults)

➲ If aged ≥65 with:
- coagulopathy – history of bleeding, clotting disorder, current anti-coagulant treatment
- dangerous mechanism of injury – a pedestrian or cyclist struck by a motor vehicle, an occupant ejected from a motor vehicle or a fall from a height of greater than 1 m or five stairs

Concussion or minor head injury (GCS score = 15)[1]

1. Record GCS score
2. Record pupil size and response
3. Consider admission if alcohol or drug intoxication and there are no appropriate support structures for safe discharge
4. Consider discharge if no indication for CT of the head
5. If discharged, supply head injury advice and leaflet as per local policy

Additional information

Glasgow Coma Scale (minimum score 3, maximum score 15)

Best motor response		Best verbal response		Eyes open	
Obeys commands	6	Orientated	5	Spontaneously	4
Localises pain	5	Confused	4	Verbal command	3
Withdraws from pain	4	Inappropriate words	3	Pain	2
Abnormal flexion	3	Incomprehensible sounds	2	No response	1
Abnormal extension	2	No vocalisations	1		
No movement	1				

Selecting patients for CT imaging of the head

Criteria for immediate request for CT scan of the head (adults)

- ➲ GCS score <13 on initial assessment in the emergency department
- ➲ GCS score <15 at 2 hours post injury on assessment in the emergency department
- ➲ Vomiting more than once
- ➲ Post-traumatic seizure
- ➲ Suspected open or depressed skull fracture
- ➲ Focal neurological deficit
- ➲ Any signs of basal skull fracture (haemotympanum, 'panda' eyes, cerebrospinal fluid leakage from the ear or nose, Battle's sign)
- ➲ Amnesia >30 minutes prior to injury

Immediate request for CT scan of the head provided patient has experienced some loss of consciousness or amnesia since the injury (adults)

➲ If aged ≥65 with:
  - coagulopathy – history of bleeding, clotting disorder, current anti-coagulant treatment
  - dangerous mechanism of injury – a pedestrian or cyclist struck by a motor vehicle, an occupant ejected from a motor vehicle or a fall from a height of greater than 1 m or five stairs

The patient should be discharged with a responsible adult and the following advice

➲ The patient should rest for 2–3 days; failure to rest may result in symptoms such as dizziness and nausea.
➲ Simple analgesia should be taken regularly to manage any symptoms.
➲ The patient should seek help if he or she experiences any persistent vomiting, increase in symptoms, confusion or seizure.

Cervical spine injury[2]

1. Establish and maintain a patent airway with adequate ventilation
2. Remove patient from spinal board or extrication device using a coordinated log roll
3. Immobilise the C-spine
4. Consider X-ray as per NEXUS (National Emergency X-Radiography Utilization Study) guidelines
5. CT imaging if indicated
6. Consider clearing C-spine

Additional information
Airway: simple airway adjuncts and suction
➲ Seek senior input in assessment if simple measures do not maintain airway
➲ Maintain oxygen saturations at 94%–98%

Immobilisation of the C-spine
➲ Manual in-line immobilisation, or
➲ Hard collar and blocks secured with tape
➲ Review neurological status and for other injuries to the spine

NEXUS low-risk criteria for determining if radiography is indicated after C-spine injury
Radiography is not recommended if a patient meets all of the following criteria:
➲ absence of tenderness at the posterior midline of the C-spine
➲ absence of a focal neurologic deficit
➲ normal level of alertness
➲ no evidence of intoxication
➲ absence of clinically apparent pain that might distract the patient from the pain of a C-spine injury.

X-ray views
➲ Anterior-posterior view
➲ Lateral view (must include C7/T1 junction)
➲ Odontoid peg view (open mouth)

CT imaging

⮞ Unable to clear C-spine using plain film

When to consider clearing C-spine

⮞ No criterion of X-ray, or
⮞ Normal X-ray in fully conscious patient, or
⮞ Normal CT in fully conscious patient

Soft tissue neck injury (whiplash)[2]

1. Consider clearing C-spine
2. Remove immobilisation
3. Assess movement
4. Consider further imaging as per local policy or clinical judgement
5. If considering further imaging, reapply immobilisation immediately

Additional information

When to consider clearing C-spine

- ➲ No criterion of X-ray (NB: NEXUS low-risk criteria), or
- ➲ Normal X-ray in fully conscious patient, or
- ➲ Normal CT in fully conscious patient

NEXUS low-risk criteria for determining if radiography is indicated after C-spine injury

Radiography is not recommended if a patient meets all of the following criteria:

- ➲ absence of tenderness at the posterior midline of the C-spine
- ➲ absence of a focal neurologic deficit
- ➲ normal level of alertness
- ➲ no evidence of intoxication
- ➲ absence of clinically apparent pain that might distract the patient from the pain of a C-spine injury.

Request patient to complete the following movements

- ➲ Slowly flex at the neck ('chin to chest')
- ➲ Slowly turn head laterally ('side to side')

Dislocation (overview)

1. Confirm nature of injury from history and likely anatomical site – document injury and describe in relation to displacement of distal bone
2. Assess neurovascular status
3. Analgesia
4. X-ray of affected area
5. Reduce dislocation as soon as possible to minimise complications, using appropriate analgesia and sedation
6. Obtain post-reduction X-ray to confirm position and review neurovascular status

Additional information

Neurovascular examination

➲ Consider immediate reduction prior to X-ray if neurovascular status not intact:
  - inform orthopaedics immediately for further input

Shoulder dislocation

1. Assess neurovascular status prior to reduction
2. Shoulder X-ray
3. Reduce dislocation with appropriate sedation and analgesia
4. Assess neurovascular status post reduction
5. Immobilise with collar and cuff
6. Obtain post-reduction X-ray

Additional information

Neurovascular examination

➲ Auxiliary nerve ('regimental badge', C5) and deltoid function
➲ Palpate for radial pulse

Shoulder X-ray

➲ Anterior-posterior and auxiliary or scapular 'Y' views:
  - confirm position of dislocation
  - ensure no coexisting fracture

Sedation and analgesia

➲ Appropriate sedation titrated to effect
➲ Titrate morphine by slow intravenous (IV) administration

Ensure full monitoring and observation and that two clinicians trained in airway management are present.

Fractured pelvis[3,4]

1. Stabilise and immobilise the pelvis as per local protocol
2. Examine pelvic region, perineum and perform rectal examination for anal tone
3. Provide adequate analgesia
4. Obtain pelvic X-ray and urinalysis to assess extent of injury
5. Venous thromboembolism prophylaxis
6. Initiate preoperative assessment

Additional information

Pelvic examination

➲ *Do not* spring or rock the pelvis

Analgesia

➲ Titrate morphine by slow IV administration

Pelvic X-ray

➲ Assess any disruption of normal pelvic contours and Shenton's line
➲ Assess for asymmetry, widening of the sacroiliac joints or pubic symphysis

Follow local venous thromboembolism policy

Note potential contraindications and act in accordance with local policy:
➲ active bleeding
➲ acquired bleeding disorders
➲ concurrent use of anticoagulants known to increase the risk of bleeding
➲ lumbar puncture, epidural, spinal anaesthesia expected within the next 12 hours
➲ lumbar puncture, epidural, spinal anaesthesia within the previous 4 hours
➲ acute stroke
➲ thrombocytopenia (platelet count less than $75 \times 10^9/L$)
➲ uncontrolled systolic hypertension
➲ untreated inherited bleeding disorders

Preoperative assessment

➲ Record coexisting morbidities, medication, mental state, mobility and functional ability
➲ Consider the following additional tests prior to admission depending on the patient's history:
  ● blood gas
  ● lung function
  ● urine analysis
  ● chest X-ray
  ● ECG

Fractured neck of femur[3-5]

1. IV access
2. Provide adequate analgesia according to local policy
3. Request appropriate imaging
4. Venous thromboembolism prophylaxis
5. Institute early pressure area care
6. Initiate preoperative assessment

Additional information

IV access

⮞ Venous bloods: FBC, U&E, INR, group and save
⮞ 1 L 0.9% saline over 6 hours

Analgesia

⮞ Titrate morphine by slow IV administration
⮞ Consider nerve blocks for additional analgesia or to limit opioid dosage

Imaging

⮞ X-ray hip and pelvis (anterior-posterior ± lateral views)
⮞ Offer magnetic resonance imaging (MRI) if hip fracture is suspected despite negative anterior-posterior pelvis and lateral hip X-rays. If MRI is not available within 24 hours or is contraindicated, consider CT

Follow local venous thromboembolism policy

Note potential contraindications and act in accordance with local policy:
⮞ active bleeding
⮞ acquired bleeding disorders
⮞ concurrent use of anticoagulants known to increase the risk of bleeding
⮞ lumbar puncture, epidural, spinal anaesthesia expected within the next 12 hours
⮞ lumbar puncture, epidural, spinal anaesthesia within the previous 4 hours
⮞ acute stroke
⮞ thrombocytopenia (platelet count less than 75×10^9/L)
⮞ uncontrolled systolic hypertension
⮞ untreated inherited bleeding disorders

Preoperative assessment

➔ Record coexisting morbidities, medication, mental state, mobility and functional ability
➔ Consider the following additional tests prior to admission depending on the patient's history:
  ● blood gas
  ● lung function
  ● urine analysis
  ● chest X-ray
  ● ECG

Fractured ankle[6]

1. Assess function and neurovascular status
2. Consider IV access
3. Provide adequate analgesia
4. Imaging as indicated by the Ottawa ankle rules
5. Disposal

If fracture confirmed:
- ➲ treat as per local policy
- ➲ seek senior and/or orthopaedic opinion.

If imaging not required or no fracture seen, discharge with advice:
- ➲ on conservative management and graduated early exercise
- ➲ to return if difficulty weight-bearing at 2 days post injury for immobilisation with plaster cast or functional brace.

Additional information

Neurovascular examination
- ➲ Consider immediate reduction prior to X-ray if neurovascular status not intact or skin at risk:
  - inform orthopaedics immediately for further input

Analgesia
- ➲ Consider titrating morphine by slow IV administration if severe pain

Ottawa ankle rules
The Ottawa ankle rules are for assessing whether an ankle X-ray series is indicated. X-rays are only required if there is any pain in the malleolar zone and any one of the following.
- ➲ Bone tenderness along the distal 6 cm of the posterior edge or tip of the medial malleolus, or
- ➲ Bone tenderness along the distal 6 cm of the posterior edge or tip of the lateral malleolus, or
- ➲ An inability to bear weight both immediately and in the emergency department

All fracture dislocations require urgent assessment and reduction to prevent further limb damage

Conservative treatment

➲ Ice, elevate, early exercise

- Non-weight-bearing movement to weight-bearing movement as tolerated

Fractured scaphoid

1. Assess function and neurovascular status
2. Provide adequate analgesia depending on severity of pain
3. X-ray
4. If radiological evidence of fracture:
   - apply scaphoid plaster cast
   - seek senior or orthopaedic advice
   - arrange fracture clinic appointment (earliest available appointment)
5. If no radiological evidence of fracture:
   - apply plaster cast or splint as per local policy
   - arrange review as per local policy
   - simple analgesia with advice

Additional information
Neurovascular examination
⊃ Inform orthopaedics immediately for further input if abnormality present

Clinical findings suggestive of scaphoid fracture
⊃ Tenderness in the anatomical snuff box
⊃ Tenderness over dorsal aspect of scaphoid
⊃ Tenderness over palmar aspect of scaphoid
⊃ Swelling over distal aspect of wrist
⊃ Tenderness or pain on thumb compression
⊃ Difficulty with gripping
⊃ Tenderness or pain with ulnar or radial deviation of wrist

Analgesia
⊃ Paracetamol 1 g ± codeine 60 mg, or
⊃ Titrate morphine by slow IV administration

Imaging
⊃ Plain X-ray scaphoid views (anterior-posterior, lateral, obliques)

Advice
⊃ Imperative that the patient returns for the review appointment
⊃ To return earlier than arranged if symptoms get worse or pain increases

Fractured distal radius

1. Assess function and neurovascular status
2. Provide adequate analgesia depending of severity of pain according to local policy
3. X-ray
4. Un-displaced fractures:
   - immobilise in plaster (backslab)
   - elevate with sling
   - discharge with analgesia and fracture clinic appointment
5. Displaced fractures:
   - reduction under regional block (following local policy)
   - post reduction:
     > immobilise in plaster
     > neurovascular assessment
     > repeat X-ray
     > advise appropriate follow-up

Additional information

Neurovascular examination

➲ Consider immediate reduction prior to X-ray if neurovascular status not intact or skin at risk:
   - inform orthopaedics immediately for further input

Test and document details

➲ Deformity
➲ Scaphoid tenderness
➲ Radial pulse
➲ Median nerve
➲ Ulnar nerve
➲ Radial nerve

Analgesia

➲ Paracetamol 1 g ± codeine 60 mg, or
➲ Titrate morphine by slow IV administration

X-ray

➲ Wrist (anterior-posterior and lateral views)

Sprain or strain

1. Obtain details from the history and perform examination of affected area
2. Provide adequate analgesia depending on severity of pain
3. Imaging is not routinely required for simple injuries
4. General principles of management
5. Discharge advice

Additional information

Key points from the history include

- Mechanism of injury
- Any similar injuries previously
- Loss of function
- Any treatment thus far
- Swelling (was this immediate?)

Analgesia

- Paracetamol 1 g ± codeine 30 mg/60 mg

X-ray may be indicted if any of the following are present

- Bony tenderness
- Swelling or bruising over a bone or joint
- Loss of function

Management

Conservative

- Ice, elevate, early exercise
  - Minimal movement to increased movement as tolerated, e.g. non-weight-bearing movement to weight-bearing movement as tolerated
- Immobilise if severe pain initially after injury or continuing pain or loss of function after 48 hours

Advice

- Recovery may take weeks (4–6 weeks on average)
- Seek advice if pain continues or loss of function is present after 48 hours
- Offer any patient information leaflets as per local policy

Laceration[7]

1. Identify and control significant bleeding with direct pressure or pressure dressing
2. Full examination of the wound
3. Obtain information surrounding the injury
4. X-rays are indicated if transfer of material or foreign body is suspected
5. Tetanus vaccine should be offered if indicated and no previous reaction noted
6. Disposal

Simple lacerations:
⊃ cleaned and closed with appropriate follow-up with general practitioner (GP) or practice nurse if required

Lacerations involving special areas (mouth, genitalia):
⊃ referral for review by appropriate specialists if required

Additional information
Haemorrhage
⊃ If significant (actual or perceived) haemorrhage, treat as hypovolaemic shock

Key points of wound examination
⊃ Location of wound
⊃ Length and depth
⊃ Tissue loss
⊃ Contamination of the wound
⊃ Exploration to exclude injury to deep structures
⊃ Assess function of underlying structures, e.g. neurovascular, tendon, ligament

Key details of wound history
Document details for possible medico-legal implications:
⊃ time of injury
⊃ what caused the injury?
⊃ other injuries

- was anybody else involved
- mechanism of injury
- tetanus status

Some types of tetanus-prone wounds

- Wounds or burns that require surgical intervention that is delayed for more than 6 hours
- Wounds or burns that show a significant degree of devitalised tissue or a puncture-type injury, particularly where there has been contact with soil or manure
- Wounds containing foreign bodies
- Compound fractures
- Wounds or burns in patients who have systemic sepsis

References

1. National Institute for Health and Clinical Excellence. *Head Injury: NICE clinical guideline 56.* London: NICE; 2007. www.nice.org.uk/CG56
2. Hoffman JR, Mower WR, Wolfson AB, *et al.* National Emergency X-Radiography Utilization Study Group. Validity of a set of clinical criteria to rule out injury to the cervical spine in patients with blunt trauma. *N Engl J Med.* 2000; **343**(2): 94–9.
3. National Institute for Health and Clinical Excellence. *Preoperative Tests: NICE clinical guideline 3.* London: NICE; 2003. www.nice.org.uk/CG3
4. National Institute for Health and Clinical Excellence. *Venous thromboembolism: NICE clinical guideline 92.* London: NICE; 2010. www.nice.org.uk/CG92
5. Scottish Intercollegiate Guidelines Network. *Management of Hip Fracture in Older People: SIGN guideline 111, Section 4: Emergency Department Management.* Edinburgh: SIGN; 2009. www.sign.ac.uk/pdf/sign111.pdf
6. Stiell IG, McKnight RG, Greenberg GH, *et al.* Implementation of the Ottawa ankle rules. *JAMA.* 1994; **271**(11): 827–32.
7. Tetanus: the green book, chapter 30: pp. 367–84. In Department of Health. *Immunisation Against Infectious Disease.* London: Department of Health; 2012 (updated 2013).

2

MEDICAL EMERGENCIES

ST elevation myocardial infarction (STEMI)

1. Confirm STEMI through ECG changes
2. **M**orphine, **O**xygen, **N**itrates, **A**spirin
3. Assess suitability for percutaneous coronary intervention (PCI) or thrombolysis
4. Review glucose levels
5. Post-resuscitation care: immediate removal to coronary care unit

Additional information

STEMI ECG changes

➲ ST elevation ≥2 mm in two or more contiguous chest leads, and/or
➲ ≥1 mm in two or more contiguous limb leads, and/or
➲ New left bundle branch block

Initial treatment

➲ **M**orphine ≤10 mg IV titrated to effect (diamorphine as an alternative)
➲ **O**xygen: ensure saturations are 94%–98%; if chronic obstructive pulmonary disease (COPD), 88%–92%
➲ **N**itrates 3–5 mg buccal or sublingual as glyceryl trinitrate (GTN)
➲ **A**spirin 300 mg chewed

PCI or thrombolysis

➲ PCI is treatment of choice for STEMI
➲ Thrombolysis (*if PCI unavailable*)

Thrombolysis contraindications

Absolute contraindications:
➲ gastrointestinal bleed within last month
➲ ischaemic stroke in last 6 months
➲ haemorrhagic stroke or stroke of unknown origin at any time
➲ major trauma, surgery or head injury within 3 weeks
➲ aortic dissection
➲ known bleeding disorder

Relative contraindications:
- current anticoagulant therapy
- transient ischaemic attack (TIA) in last 6 months
- pregnancy or within 1 week post-partum
- traumatic resuscitation
- refractory hypertension (systolic >180 mmHg)

Glucose
- If glucose >10, start to treat with insulin sliding scale

Acute coronary syndrome[1]

1. Exclude STEMI through ECG changes
2. **M**orphine, **O**xygen, **N**itrates, **A**spirin
3. Assess cardiac markers
4. Review glucose levels
5. Admission for further medical assessment and management

Additional information

STEMI ECG changes

⊃ ST elevation ≥2 mm in two or more contiguous chest leads, and/or
⊃ ≥1 mm in two or more contiguous limb leads, and/or
⊃ New left bundle branch block

Initial treatment

Start management of acute coronary syndrome as soon as suspected.

⊃ **M**orphine: titrate by slow IV administration (diamorphine as an alternative)
⊃ **O**xygen: ensure saturations are 94%–98%; if COPD, 88%–92%
⊃ **N**itrates 3–5 mg buccal or sublingual as GTN
⊃ **A**spirin 300 mg chewed

Consider:

⊃ clopidogrel 300 mg orally
⊃ low-molecular-weight heparin 1 mg/kg subcutaneously

Cardiac markers

⊃ Troponin negative: unstable angina or non-cardiac pain
⊃ Troponin positive: non-ST elevation myocardial infarction (NSTEMI)

Glucose

⊃ If glucose >10, start treatment with insulin sliding scale

Acute heart failure or pulmonary oedema

1. Resuscitation as required
2. Bloods
3. Investigations: chest X-ray, ECG
4. If systolic >90 administer:
   - two puffs of GTN
   - diamorphine 1 mg IV (repeat up to 5 mg)
   - furosemide 40–80 mg IV (repeat up to 120 mg)
5. If patient does not improve with the above medication consider:
   - GTN IV (50 mg in 50 mL 0.9 % saline at 2–10 mL/hour)
   - Titrate GTN to ensure systolic ≥90 mmHg
6. If life-threatening, gain early specialist advice and support

Additional information

Resuscitation

- ➔ Oxygen: ensure saturations are 94%–98%; if COPD, 88%–92%
- ➔ IV access

Blood tests

- ➔ Arterial blood gas
- ➔ Venous: FBC, U&E, LFTs, CRP, glucose, troponin I, CK, BNP
- ➔ Blood cultures if temperature ≥38.0°C

Additional considerations

- ➔ Catheterisation
- ➔ Continuous positive airway pressure
- ➔ High dependency unit or ITU intervention
- ➔ Central venous pressure (CVP) monitoring

Tachycardia

1. Resuscitation as required
2. Assess adverse signs
3. If unstable – adverse signs present:
   - synchronised DC shocks (up to three attempts); ensure adequate sedation and analgesia are utilised

   If unsuccessful
   - amiodarone 300 mg IV over 10–20 minutes and then repeat shocks
   - maintenance – amiodarone 900 mg over 24 hours
4. If stable and regular broad complex tachycardia
   - amiodarone 300 mg IV over 20–60 minutes
   - if previous supraventricular tachycardia with bundle branch block, administer adenosine 6 mg IV bolus
5. If torsade de pointes:
   - magnesium 2 g IV over 10 minutes
6. If stable and *regular* narrow complex tachycardia:
   - vagal manoeuvres
   - if ineffective, adenosine 6 mg rapid IV bolus; if ineffective then adenosine 12 mg IV and flush
   - monitor ECG continuously

   If stable and *irregular* narrow complex tachycardia:
   - digoxin 500 mcg, or metoprolol 5 mg if <48 hours since onset, or
   - amiodarone 300 mg IV 20–60 minutes, then 900 mg over 24 hours

Additional information

Resuscitation
- Oxygen: ensure saturations are 94%–98%; if COPD, 88%–92%
- IV access

Adverse signs
- Reduced consciousness
- Systolic <90 mmHg
- Chest pain
- Heart failure

Bradycardia

1. Resuscitation as required
2. Assess adverse signs
3. If an adverse sign is present:
   - atropine 500 mcg IV (repeat up to a maximum of 3 mg)
4. If risk of asystole then consider:
   - adrenaline 2–10 mcg/minute IV, or
   - pace transcutaneously
5. If patient deteriorates get senior help

Additional information

Resuscitation

- ⮞ Oxygen: ensure saturations are 94%–98%; if COPD, 88%–92%
- ⮞ IV access

Adverse signs

- ⮞ Reduced consciousness
- ⮞ Systolic <90 mmHg
- ⮞ Chest pain
- ⮞ Heart failure

Atropine administration

- ⮞ A patient must be continuously monitored even if an increase in heart rate (HR) is seen

Risks of asystole

- ⮞ Recent asystole
- ⮞ Mobitz II atrioventricular block
- ⮞ Complete heart block with broad QRS
- ⮞ Ventricular pause > 3 seconds

Consider alternative drugs

- ➲ Aminophylline
- ➲ Isoprenaline
- ➲ Dopamine
- ➲ Glucagon (if beta blocker or calcium channel blocker overdose)
- ➲ Glycopyrrolate instead of atropine
- ➲ Review *British National Formulary* for all individual doses

Post–cardiac arrest care[2]

1. Resuscitation as required
2. Continuous reassessment and physiological monitoring
3. Bloods
4. Investigations: chest X-ray, ECG
5. Nasogastric (NG) tube
6. Immediate transfer to ITU or coronary care unit, or
   Consider Do Not Attempt Cardiopulmonary Resuscitation documentation

Additional information

Resuscitation

- Supportive ventilation as appropriate
- Oxygen: ensure saturations are 94%–98%
- IV access if not present

Blood tests

- Arterial blood gas
- Venous – FBC, U&E, LFTs, magnesium, Ca^{2+}, glucose, troponin:
  - maintain potassium (K^+) at 4.0–4.5 mmol/L
- Blood cultures if temperature ≥38.0°C
- Blood glucose (capillary):
  - ensure tight blood glucose levels are maintained (≤10 mmol/L), using an insulin sliding scale

Rationale for investigations

- Arterial blood gas: use as an immediate marker for K^+ levels and acid base status
- ECG: view recent ECG changes or use as a baseline
- Chest X-ray: exclude fractured ribs and pneumothorax, or establish position of any tubes or lines

Prior to ITU transfer

- Consider induction of internal/external cooling as per local policy

Asthma[3]

1. Assess severity
2. Oxygen administration
3. Bloods
4. Continuous reassessment and physiological monitoring
5. Consider admission depending on severity

If acute severe or life-threatening:
1. administer treatment and investigate as per asthma care bundle
2. if life-threatening, gain senior support and ITU advice immediately
3. prednisolone 40–50 mg oral or hydrocortisone 100 mg IV
4. consider IV magnesium 1.2–2 g if no initial response to acute severe asthma with bronchodilator therapy
5. consider chest X-ray if concerned about possible pneumothorax or infective or pneumonia exacerbation

Additional information

Asthma severity

Moderate

⮞ Increasing symptoms
⮞ Peak expiratory flow rate (PEFR) >50%–75% of best or predicted
⮞ No features of acute severe asthma

Acute severe

Any one of:
⮞ PEFR 33%–50% of best or predicted
⮞ Respiratory rate ≥25 breaths per minute
⮞ Pulse ≥110 beats per minute
⮞ Inability to complete sentences in one breath

Life-threatening (acute severe + one of the following)

⮞ Altered conscious level
⮞ PEFR <33% of best or predicted
⮞ SpO_2 <92%
⮞ PaO_2 <8 kPa
⮞ Normal $PaCO_2$

- Silent chest
- Poor respiratory effort
- Exhaustion
- Cyanosis
- Hypotension
- Arrhythmia

Oxygen administration
- Recommended target saturation range is 94%–98%
- Administer nebulisers under pressure of oxygen to maintain saturation
- Nebulised salbutamol 5 mg prn:
  - if moderate asthma administer salbutamol inhaler (four puffs initially, then two puffs every 2 minutes to a maximum of 10) via a spacer
- Nebulised ipratropium bromide 500 mcg (every 4–6 hours)

Blood tests
- Arterial blood gas if indicated
- Venous: FBC, U&E, CRP
- Measure theophylline level if part of normal prescription
- Blood cultures if temperature ≥38.0°C

Community-acquired pneumonia[4,5]

1. Assess severity
2. Oxygen administration
3. Bloods
4. Investigations: chest X-ray, ECG, sputum for culture if productive cough
5. Empirical antibiotic treatment referenced to severity

Additional information
Assessing severity of pneumonia
1 point for each

- ⮑ **C**onfusion (new onset)
- ⮑ **U**rea >7 mmol/L
- ⮑ **R**espiratory rate >30
- ⮑ **B**lood pressure (BP) (systolic <90)
- ⮑ **A**ge ≥**65**

Mild 0–1 (often managed at home)
Moderate 2 (hospital admission)
Severe ≥3 (high dependency unit or ITU input required)

Oxygen administration
- ⮑ Ensure saturations are 94%–98%; if COPD, 88%–92%

Blood tests
- ⮑ Arterial blood gas
- ⮑ Venous: FBC, U&E, LFTs, CRP
- ⮑ Blood cultures if temperature ≥38.0°C

Empirical antibiotic treatment
- ⮑ Mild – amoxicillin 500 mg tds
- ⮑ Moderate – amoxicillin 500 mg tds:
    - if oral administration not possible, amoxicillin 500 mg tds IV
- ⮑ Severe – co-amoxiclav 1.2 g tds IV and clarithromycin 500 mg bd IV

Antibiotics and admission depend on local policy. Ensure a full review of local policy is undertaken if the patient has any allergy.

Pneumothorax[6]

Primary pneumothorax

1. Sit patient up and administer 100% oxygen
2. Bloods: arterial blood gas if dyspnoea present
3. Expiratory chest X-ray
4. If short of breath and rim of air >2 cm on chest X-ray aspirate:
   - re-aspirate if required
   - if aspiration not successful insert a chest drain
5. Once stable, reduce the oxygen dose and aim for target saturation range of 94%–98%

Secondary pneumothorax

1. Sit patient up and administer 100% oxygen
2. Bloods: arterial blood gas if dyspnoea present
3. Expiratory chest X-ray
4. If short of breath, aged over 50 and rim of air >2 cm on chest X-ray, insert a chest drain
5. If minimally breathless, aged under 50 and rim of air <2 cm on chest X-ray then consider aspiration:
   - if aspiration unsuccessful then insert a chest drain
   - if successful then admit to hospital and observe for 24 hours
6. Once stable, reduce the oxygen dose and aim for a target saturation range of 94%–98%; if COPD, 88%–92%

Tension pneumothorax

1. Sit patient up and administer 100% oxygen
2. Treat prior to chest X-ray
3. Insert a large bore cannula into the second intercostal space in the mid-clavicular line
4. Insert a large bore chest drain
5. Chest X-ray
6. Once stable, reduce the oxygen dose and aim for a target saturation range of 94%–98%; if COPD, 88%–92%

Deep vein thrombosis[7]

1. Assess clinical probability using the Wells Score prior to any test
2. Bloods
3. Investigations: chest X-ray if any breathlessness, ECG, consider proximal leg vein ultrasound if available
4. Analgesia
5. Start treatment dose low-molecular-weight heparin anticoagulation in accordance with local policy

Additional information

Wells score: clinical probability

+1 point each

⮩ Active cancer (including treatment within last 6 months)
⮩ Paralysis, paresis or recent plaster immobilisation of the leg
⮩ Bedridden for more than 3 days or major surgery requiring general anaesthesia in the last 12 weeks
⮩ Local tenderness along veins
⮩ Whole leg swollen:
  - >3 cm calf swelling (when compared with asymptomatic leg)
⮩ Pitting oedema confined to the symptomatic leg
⮩ Non varicose collateral superficial veins

−2 points

⮩ Alternative diagnosis equally likely as deep vein thrombosis (DVT)

Score

≥2: DVT likely
≤1: DVT unlikely

If DVT is suspected and shown as *likely* on the two-level DVT Wells score:
⮩ complete a proximal leg vein ultrasound scan
⮩ if unavailable, then administer parenteral anticoagulant until proximal leg vein ultrasound scan completed.

If DVT is suspected and shown as *unlikely* on the two-level DVT Wells score:
⮩ undertake a D-dimer test.

If D-dimer positive:

➲ complete a proximal leg vein ultrasound scan
➲ if unavailable, then administer an interim 24-hour dose of a parenteral anticoagulant.

In all cases arrange a review as per local policy.

Blood tests

➲ Arterial blood gas if patient is short of breath
➲ Venous: FBC, U&E, CRP, clotting screen, D-dimer

Analgesia

➲ Paracetamol 1 g ± codeine 60 mg, or
➲ Titrate morphine by slow IV administration

Pulmonary embolus[5,7]

1. Assess clinical probability of pulmonary embolus (PE)
2. Resuscitation as required
3. Analgesia
4. Bloods
5. Investigations: chest X-ray, ECG, consider CT pulmonary angiogram (CTPA)

Additional information

Wells score: clinical probability for pulmonary embolus

Clinically suspected DVT	3.0 points
Alternative diagnosis is less likely than PE	3.0 points
HR >100	1.5 points
Immobilisation or surgery in previous 4 weeks	1.5 points
History of DVT or PE	1.5 points
Haemoptysis	1.0 points
Malignancy (treatment for within 6 months, palliative)	1.0 points

Scores: >4 PE likely; ≤4 PE unlikely

➲ If PE is suspected with a likely two-level PE Wells score
  ● CTPA to confirm diagnosis
  ● administer interim parenteral anticoagulant therapy if a CTPA cannot be carried out immediately
➲ If PE is suspected with an unlikely two-level PE Wells score, complete a D-dimer test
  ● If D-dimer positive:
    ❭ CTPA to confirm diagnosis
    ❭ administer interim parenteral anticoagulant therapy if a CTPA cannot be carried out immediately

Resuscitation

➲ Oxygen: ensure saturations are 94%–98%
➲ IV access
➲ Fluid resuscitate if BP <90 systolic:
  ● consider thrombolytic therapy for patients with PE and haemodynamic instability

Analgesia

⮕ Paracetamol 1 g ± codeine 60 mg, or
⮕ Titrate morphine by slow IV administration

Blood tests

⮕ Arterial blood gas (repeat as required):
  • if pH <7.35, get early senior or ITU support as required
⮕ Venous: FBC, U&E, CRP, clotting screen, D-dimer

Investigations

⮕ ECG – may see sinus tachycardia, right bundle branch block or SI QIII TIII

Chronic obstructive pulmonary disease[8,9]

1. Oxygen
2. Bloods
3. Investigations: chest X-ray, ECG, sputum for culture if productive cough
4. Nebulisers:
   - if no response to nebulisers consider –
     › theophylline IV
     › prednisolone 40 mg oral or hydrocortisone 200 mg IV
5. Antibiotics if evidence of infection
6. Consider non-invasive ventilation if hypercapnia persists

Additional information

Oxygen

➲ Start oxygen therapy at 24%–28% via venturi mask
➲ Titrate to maintain oxygen saturations 88%–92%

Blood tests

➲ Arterial blood gas (repeat as required):
  - if pH <7.35, get early senior or ITU support as required
➲ Venous: FBC, U&E, CRP
➲ Measure theophylline level if part of normal prescription
➲ Blood cultures if temperature ≥38.0°C

Rationale for investigations

➲ Chest X-ray: exclude infection, pneumothorax and other causes
➲ ECG: exclude co-morbidity

Nebulisers

➲ Salbutamol 5 mg as required
➲ Ipratropium bromide 500 mcg

If acidosis or hypercapnia present, nebulisers should be delivered by compressed air

Empirical antibiotics

⮕ Oral: co-amoxiclav 625 mg tds or erythromycin 500 mg qds
⮕ IV: co-amoxiclav 1.2 g tds IV or erythromycin 25–50 mg/kg divided as qds

Antibiotics and admission are dependent on local policy.

Non-invasive ventilation

⮕ Ensure a clear plan is documented in case of deterioration

Type 1 respiratory failure

1. Treat underlying cause
2. Oxygen
3. Bloods
4. Investigations: chest X-ray, ECG, sputum for culture if productive cough
5. Continuous reassessment and physiological monitoring

Additional information

Respiratory failure

➲ Type 1: PaO_2 of <8 kPa with a normal or low $PaCO_2$
➲ Type 2: PaO_2 of <8 kPa and a $PaCO_2$ of >6 kPa

Treat underlying cause

➲ If due to infection, administer antibiotics according to local policy

Oxygen

➲ 35%–60% using a venturi mask

Blood tests

➲ Arterial blood gas
➲ Venous: FBC, U&E, CRP
➲ Blood cultures if temperature ≥38.0°C

Monitoring

➲ If poor or inadequate response, contact senior or ITU support as required

Type 2 respiratory failure[9]

1. Treat underlying cause if possible
2. Oxygen
3. Bloods
4. Investigations: chest X-ray, ECG, sputum for culture if productive cough
5. Continuous reassessment and physiological monitoring
6. If no response, contact senior or ITU support as required

Additional information

Respiratory failure

⮞ Type 1: PaO_2 of <8 kPa with a normal or low $PaCO_2$
⮞ Type 2: PaO_2 of <8 kPa and a $PaCO_2$ of >6 kPa

Oxygen

⮞ Initiate oxygen therapy at 24% via a venturi mask

Blood tests

⮞ Arterial blood gas:
  - recheck arterial blood gas after 30 minutes –
    ❯ if P_aCO_2 same or lower, increase oxygen to 28%
    ❯ if P_aCO_2 >6 kPa and P_aO_2 <8 kPa then consider non-invasive ventilation or doxapram 1.5 mg per minute IV (increased to 4 mg per minute if required)
⮞ Venous: FBC, U&E, CRP
⮞ Blood cultures if temperature ≥38.0°C

Non-invasive ventilation

Indications

⮞ COPD with a respiratory acidosis – pH <7.35 (H^+ >45 nmol/L)
⮞ Hypercapnic respiratory failure secondary to chest wall deformity (scoliosis, thoracoplasty) or neuromuscular diseases
⮞ Cardiogenic pulmonary oedema unresponsive to continuous positive airway pressure
⮞ Weaning from tracheal intubation

Not indicated in

⊃ Impaired consciousness; coma; confusion; claustrophobia

⊃ Respiratory complications – severe hypoxaemia; copious respiratory secretions; active tuberculosis; undrained pneumothorax; focal consolidation on chest X-ray; fixed upper airway obstruction

⊃ Surgical complications – vomiting/bowel obstruction; facial trauma; oesophageal surgery

⊃ Haemodynamic instability

Gastrointestinal haemorrhage (upper)[10]

1. Resuscitation as required
2. Identify risk using the Blatchford score
3. Bloods
4. Investigations: chest X-ray, ECG
5. Correct any clotting abnormalities
6. Continuous reassessment and physiological monitoring

Additional information

Resuscitation

- Oxygen: ensure saturations are 94%–98%; if COPD, 88%–92%
- IV access
- Fluid resuscitate if BP <90 systolic:
  - if patient is haemodynamically unstable –
    - contact endoscopy
    - consider Terlipressin to patients with suspected variceal bleeding at presentation (administer in accordance with local policy)
- If vomiting: nil by mouth (NBM), NG tube
- Transfuse patients with massive bleeding with blood, platelets and clotting factors in line with local protocols for managing massive bleeding

Blood tests

- Arterial blood gas as indicated
- Venous: FBC, U&E, LFTs, clotting, glucose
- X-match for six units

Correct clotting abnormalities

- Vitamin K or clotting factors or fresh frozen plasma in accordance with local policy

Monitoring

- Catheterise and monitor hourly output
- Consider central venous pressure (CVP) monitoring
- Consider ITU or anaesthetic input if patient deteriorating

Blatchford score (any score >0 is a risk of requiring an intervention)

Blatchford score admission marker	Score component value
Blood urea (mmol/L)	
×6.5 <8.0	2
×8.0 <10.0	3
×10.0 <25	4
×25	6
Haemoglobin (g/L) for men	
×120 <130	1
×100 <120	3
<100	6
Haemoglobin (g/L) for women	
×100 <120	1
<100	6
Systolic BP (mmHg)	
100–109	1
90–99	2
<90	3
Other markers	
Pulse ×100 (per minute)	1
Presentation with melaena	1
Presentation with syncope	2
Hepatic disease	2
Cardiac failure	2

Headache (general management)[11,12]

1. Establish GCS score
2. Assess for red flag symptoms
3. Analgesia
4. Bloods
5. Reassess and monitor physiology regularly
6. Once diagnosis is made follow specific protocol

Additional information

Glasgow Coma Scale (minimum score 3, maximum score 15)

Best motor response		Best verbal response		Eyes open	
Obeys commands	6	Orientated	5	Spontaneously	4
Localises pain	5	Confused	4	Verbal command	3
Withdraws from pain	4	Inappropriate words	3	Pain	2
Abnormal flexion	3	Incomprehensible sounds	2	No response	1
Abnormal extension	2	No vocalisations	1		
No movement	1				

If reduced GCS score, consider:
➲ CT of the head
➲ lumbar puncture
➲ electroencephalogram to rule out encephalitis
➲ urgent ITU input if GCS score ≤8.

Red flag symptoms
➲ New onset or change in headache in patients who are aged over 50
➲ Thunderclap: rapid time to peak headache intensity (seconds to 5 minutes)
➲ Focal neurological symptoms (e.g. limb weakness, aura <5 minutes of >1 hour)
➲ Non-focal neurological disturbance (e.g. cognitive disturbance, personality)
➲ Change in headache frequency, characteristics or associated symptoms
➲ Headache precipitated by physical exertion or Valsalva manoeuvre
➲ Headache that changes with posture
➲ New-onset headache in a patient with HIV

- New-onset headache in a patient with a history of cancer
- Patients with risk factors for cerebral venous sinus thrombosis
- Fever
- Recent (usually within the past 3 months) head trauma
- Neck stiffness
- Symptoms and signs of acute narrow-angle glaucoma
- Visual disturbance
- Reduced level of consciousness
- Jaw claudication

Consider further investigations if acute onset and:
- a history of malignancy known to metastasise to the brain
- vomiting without other obvious cause
- compromised immunity.

Analgesia
- Paracetamol 1 g ± ibuprofen 400 mg, or
- Titrate morphine by slow IV administration

Blood tests
- Arterial blood gas
- Venous: FBC, U&E, LFTs, CRP, erythrocyte sedimentation rate (ESR), glucose, clotting
- Blood cultures if temperature ≥38.0°C

Seizure and status epilepticus[13]

1. Secure airway
2. Control seizure
3. Resuscitation as required
4. Bloods
5. When seizure has stopped and if alcoholism or malnourished:
   - administer Pabrinex two pairs IV over 10 minutes
   - chlordiazepoxide 30–40 mg oral
6. Investigations

Additional information

Airway
⮕ Oxygen: 100% initially, then ensure saturations are 94%–98%; if COPD, 88%–92%
⮕ Place in recovery position

Control seizure
⮕ IV glucose (100 mL of 20%, 200 mL of 10%) if hypoglycaemia is possible or confirmed

Anticonvulsants
⮕ First line: lorazepam 4 mg IV at 2 mg per minute; repeat after 10 minutes if required:
   - rectal diazepam 10–20 mg if no IV access; repeat up to 30 mg
⮕ Second line: phenytoin 15 mg/kg IV diluted to 10 mg/mL in 0.9% sodium chloride over 20 minutes; *maintenance* – 100 mg IV tds or qds

Refractory status
⮕ Consider general anaesthesia with assisted ventilation; call for senior or ITU support

Resuscitation
⮕ IV access
⮕ Fluid resuscitate if BP <90 systolic

Blood tests

➲ Glucose level (capillary)
➲ Arterial blood gas as indicated
➲ Venous: FBC, U&E, LFTs, Ca^{2+}, magnesium, glucose, serum anticonvuls-
   ant levels
➲ Blood cultures if temperature ≥38.0°C

Investigations

➲ Urinalysis
➲ Consider CT of the brain and lumbar puncture, depending on history
➲ Consider electroencephalographic monitoring in refractory status or dia-
   gnosis in doubt (? pseudostatus)

Stroke[14]

1. Resuscitation as required
2. Contact acute stroke team if present in hospital for consideration of thrombolysis
3. Bloods
4. Investigations: consider immediate CT or MRI
5. Reassess and monitor physiology regularly
6. Admit to specialist stroke ward

Additional information

Resuscitation

- Secure airway
- Oxygen: only indicated in patients with an acute stroke if saturations <95%
- IV access
- Fluid resuscitate if BP <90 systolic
- NBM until bedside swallow screen (within 24 hours)

Glasgow Coma Scale (minimum score 3, maximum score 15)

Best motor response		Best verbal response		Eyes open	
Obeys commands	6	Orientated	5	Spontaneously	4
Localises pain	5	Confused	4	Verbal command	3
Withdraws from pain	4	Inappropriate words	3	Pain	2
Abnormal flexion	3	Incomprehensible sounds	2	No response	1
Abnormal extension	2	No vocalisations	1		
No movement	1				

Blood tests

- Venous: FBC, U&E, LFTs, clotting, glucose
- Glucose capillary:
  - maintain blood glucose between 4 and 11 mmol/L

Perform brain imaging immediately if any of the following apply

- on anticoagulant treatment
- a known bleeding tendency
- a depressed level of consciousness (GCS <13)

- ⊃ unexplained progressive or fluctuating symptoms
- ⊃ papilloedema, neck stiffness or fever
- ⊃ severe headache at onset of stroke symptoms

For patients who have had a *primary intracerebral haemorrhage excluded by brain imaging*:
- ⊃ administer aspirin 300 mg orally if they are not dysphagic; rectally or enteral tube if dysphagic
- ⊃ review allergies and history of dyspepsia – treat according to local guidelines

For patients who have had a *primary intracerebral haemorrhage confirmed*:
- ⊃ review history of anticoagulation medications and INR levels
- ⊃ normalise INR levels using a combination of prothrombin complex concentrate and intravenous vitamin K

Transient ischaemic attack[14]

1. Assess GCS score
2. Oxygen if required
3. Bloods
4. Investigations: chest X-ray, ECG
5. Assess risk of stroke using ABCD^2 score

Additional information

Glasgow Coma Scale (minimum score 3, maximum score 15)

Best motor response		Best verbal response		Eyes open	
Obeys commands	6	Orientated	5	Spontaneously	4
Localises pain	5	Confused	4	Verbal command	3
Withdraws from pain	4	Inappropriate words	3	Pain	2
Abnormal flexion	3	Incomprehensible sounds	2	No response	1
Abnormal extension	2	No vocalisations	1		
No movement	1				

➲ Ensure full resolution of stroke symptoms

Oxygen

➲ Administer 100% initially, then ensure saturations are 94%–98%; if COPD, 88%–92%

Blood tests

➲ Venous: FBC, U&E, LFTs, clotting, glucose
➲ Glucose capillary

ABCD^2 assessment when TIA suspected

A	Age: ×60 years (1 point)
B	BP: ×140/90 mmHg (1 point)
C	Clinical features: unilateral weakness (2 points), speech impairment without weakness (1 point)
D	Duration: >60 minutes (2 points); 10–59 minutes (1 point)
D	Diabetes (1 point)

Tool interpretation: ≥4 = *High* risk; <4 = *Low* risk; Maximum score = 7

- Admit all high-risk patients
- Admit or discharge all low-risk patients depending on local policy:
  - arrange specialist assessment within 1 week
- Administer 300 mg aspirin PO or anticoagulation therapy as soon as possible in accordance with local guidelines
- Patients with crescendo TIA (two or more TIAs in a week) should be treated as 'high risk'

Subarachnoid haemorrhage[15]

1. Ensure patent airway if GCS score is reduced
2. Resuscitation as required
3. Analgesia
4. Bloods
5. Investigations
6. Reassess and monitor physiology regularly

Additional information

Glasgow Coma Scale (minimum score 3, maximum score 15)

Best motor response		Best verbal response		Eyes open	
Obeys commands	6	Orientated	5	Spontaneously	4
Localises pain	5	Confused	4	Verbal command	3
Withdraws from pain	4	Inappropriate words	3	Pain	2
Abnormal flexion	3	Incomprehensible sounds	2	No response	1
Abnormal extension	2	No vocalisations	1		
No movement	1				

➲ Oxygen: ensure saturations are 94%–98%
➲ Urgent ITU input if GCS score ≤8

Resuscitation

➲ IV access
➲ Fluid resuscitate if BP <90 systolic

Analgesia

➲ Paracetamol 1 g ± codeine 60 mg, or
➲ Titrate morphine by slow IV administration

Blood tests

➲ Arterial blood gas if GCS score ≤8
➲ Venous: FBC, U&E, CRP, ESR, clotting

Investigations

⊃ Urgent CT scan of the head prior to neurosurgical opinion ('urgent' is considered as soon as possible)

⊃ Lumbar puncture for xanthochromia after 12 hours of onset of headache if CT scan is normal and a strong suspicion remains

Meningitis

1. Resuscitation as required
2. Bloods
3. Investigations
4. If clinical suspicion of bacterial meningitis administer antibiotics
5. Full clinical review for complications

Additional information

Resuscitation

➲ Oxygen: ensure saturations are 94%–98%
➲ IV access
➲ Fluid resuscitate if BP <90 systolic
➲ Fluids depending on dehydration status + normal maintenance

Blood tests

➲ Arterial blood gas as indicated
➲ Venous: FBC, U&E, LFTs, CRP, INR, glucose, viral serology, syphilis serology
➲ Blood cultures if temperature ≥38.0°C
➲ Blood glucose (capillary)

Investigations

➲ Lumbar puncture:
  • cerebrospinal fluid microscopy, white cell count and differential, protein levels, glucose, Ziehl–Neelsen (tuberculosis) and Indian ink stain (cryptococcal infection) if immunocompromised
➲ CT head scan prior to lumbar puncture if mass lesion or increased intracranial pressure suspected

Antibiotics

➲ Cefotaxime or ceftriaxone 2 g IV qds
➲ Add ampicillin 2 g 4-hourly if risk of *Listeria* (elderly, immunocompromised):
  • antibiotics and admission dependent on local policy
➲ Obtain early senior or ITU advice if signs of septicaemia

Clinical review to include

- ➲ Increased intracranial pressure
- ➲ Hydrocephalus
- ➲ Seizures
- ➲ Focal neurology

Acute renal failure

1. Resuscitation as required
2. Stop any contraindicated drugs
3. Bloods
4. Investigations: chest X-ray; ECG; microscopy, culture and sensitivity (MC&S); osmolality; urinalysis; ultrasound scan (USS)
5. Treat for high potassium if required
6. Continuous reassessment and physiological monitoring

Additional information

Resuscitation

⮕ Oxygen: ensure saturations are 94%–98%
⮕ IV access
⮕ Fluid resuscitate if BP <90 systolic
⮕ Fluid challenge if dehydrated:
  - 500 mL 0.9% sodium chloride over 30 minutes
⮕ If fluid overloaded, 40–80 mg furosemide IV STAT

Contraindicated drugs

⮕ Non-steroidal anti-inflammatory drugs, ACE inhibitors

Blood tests

⮕ Arterial blood gas
⮕ Venous: FBC, U&E, LFTs, Ca^{2+}, PO_4^{3-}, CK, CRP, ESR, INR, osmolality, LDH, autoantibodies
⮕ Blood cultures if temperature ≥38.0°C

Treatment for hyperkalaemia

⮕ If K^+ <6.5 mmol/L, 15 g calcium resonium qds PO
⮕ If K^+ ≥6.5, insulin sliding scale
⮕ If ECG changes are noted, administer 10 mL of 10% calcium gluconate IV
⮕ Treatment may differ depending on local policy

Monitoring

➲ Catheterise and monitor hourly output

➲ Consider CVP monitoring

➲ Consider dialysis if:

- hyperkalaemia ≥7
- pH ≤7
- pulmonary oedema that is not resolving
- pericarditis
- reduced GCS score

➲ Consider ITU or anaesthetic input if patient deteriorating

Urinary tract infection[16]

1. Resuscitation as required
2. Bloods
3. Investigations: urinalysis
4. Antibiotic treatment
5. Consider admission
6. If discharged advise to attend GP

Additional information

Resuscitation

- ⇒ Oxygen: ensure saturations are 94%–98%; if COPD, 88%–92%
- ⇒ IV access
- ⇒ Fluid resuscitate if BP <90 systolic

Blood tests

- ⇒ Venous: FBC, U&E, CRP
- ⇒ Blood cultures if temperature ≥38°C

Urinalysis

- ⇒ Use urinalysis to support diagnosis of urinary tract infection (UTI)
- ⇒ Treat empirically if positive for two of nitrites, leukocytes, haematuria or proteinuria:
  - midstream specimen of urine for MC&S if strong suspicion of UTI
- ⇒ Do not use urinalysis to diagnose a UTI in catheterised patients

Antibiotic treatment

- ⇒ *Cystitis*: trimethoprim 200 mg PO bd
- ⇒ Second line: co-amoxiclav 625 mg PO tds
- ⇒ *Upper UTI*: ciprofloxacin 500 mg PO bd, or co-amoxiclav 625 mg PO tds
- ⇒ *Prostatitis*: ciprofloxacin 500 mg PO bd

Antibiotics are dependent on local policy.

Duration of antibiotic course

➲ Simple infection: 3 days
➲ Complicated infection: 5–10 days (upper UTI, male, renal disease, systemically unwell)

When to consider admission of patient

➲ Sepsis
➲ Acute pyelonephritis
➲ Requires IV antibiotics or fluid replacement
➲ Request urologist advice in men who have upper UTI, have failed to respond to antibiotics, have had recurrent UTIs

Inform patient's GP if any of the following is outstanding

➲ Midstream specimen of urine result – treatment regimen may be modified in light of culture results
➲ Referral for investigations in all: male patients, recurrent infections in female patients, pregnancy, renal impairment

Diabetic ketoacidosis[17]

1. Resuscitation as required
2. Bloods
3. Investigations: ECG, urinalysis
4. Insulin sliding scale regimen as per local policy
5. Continuous reassessment and physiological monitoring as indicated

Additional information

Resuscitation

⮞ Oxygen: ensure saturations are 94%–98%; if COPD, 88%–92%
⮞ IV access
⮞ Fluid regimen as per local policy
  • Potassium replacement should be initiated early with regular monitoring for hypokalaemia

Blood tests

⮞ Arterial blood gas (get senior help if pH <7.0)
⮞ Venous: FBC, U&E, CRP, amylase, glucose, HbA_{1c}, bicarbonate, osmolality
  • osmolality = {2 (Na + K) + urea + glucose}
⮞ Blood cultures if temperature ≥38°C
⮞ Blood glucose (capillary):
  • administer six units soluble insulin IV if >20 mmol/L

Urinalysis

⮞ Consider HONK if no ketonuria present

Monitoring

⮞ Catheterise and monitor hourly output
⮞ NG tube
⮞ Consider ITU or anaesthetic input if patient deteriorating

Hyperglycaemic hyperosmolar non-ketosis[18]

1. Resuscitation as required
2. Bloods
3. Investigations: ECG, urinalysis
4. Insulin sliding scale regimen as per local policy
5. Start treatment dose of low-molecular-weight heparin according to weight and local policy
6. Continuous reassessment and physiological monitoring as indicated

Additional information

Resuscitation

➲ Oxygen: ensure saturations are 94%–98%; if COPD, 88%–92%
➲ IV access
➲ Fluid regimen as per local policy

Blood tests

➲ Arterial blood gas (if acidosis consider diabetic ketoacidosis)
➲ Venous: FBC, U&E, CRP, glucose, HbA$_{1c}$, bicarbonate, osmolality
  • osmolality = {2 (Na + K) + urea + glucose}
➲ Blood cultures if temperature ≥38°C
➲ Blood glucose (capillary):
  • give six units soluble insulin IV if >20 mmol/L

Urinalysis

➲ Consider diabetic ketoacidosis if ketonuria present

Monitoring

➲ Catheterise and monitor hourly output
➲ NG tube
➲ Consider ITU or anaesthetic input if patient deteriorating

Hypoglycaemia[19]

If GCS score = 15

1. Administer Glucogel or equivalent
2. Give slowly digested starchy carbohydrate food to maintain glucose levels
3. Assess capillary glucose every 15 minutes and maintain >4 mmol/L
4. If no response – reconsider diagnosis and get senior help
5. Consider discharge if patient fits criterion

If low GCS score or in coma

1. Resuscitation as required
2. IV glucose STAT (100 mL of 20%, 200 mL of 10%)
3. If hypoglycaemia is the cause, then GCS score should return to normal in 5–10 minutes.
4. If patient does not respond, reconsider diagnosis
5. Get senior help or ITU if patient does not return to a GCS score of 15
6. Consider discharge if patient fits criteria

Additional information if GCS score = 15

Criteria for discharge

- Returned to baseline level of functioning
- No evidence of concurrent illness
- Capillary blood glucose ≥4 mmol/L

Additional information if low GCS score or in coma

Resuscitation

- Oxygen: ensure saturations are 94%–98%
- IV access
- Secondary survey to rule out other cause

Consider insulin overdose

- If insulin overdose noted, administer 1 mg glucagon SC, IM, IV (not to be given to patients under the influence of alcohol, known alcoholics, emaciated patients or patients in a state of starvation)

Continued treatment

➲ Maintain glucose >5 mmol/L
➲ Administer 1000 mL 10% IV glucose over 6 hours
➲ Monitor capillary glucose levels every 30 minutes

Altered level of consciousness or coma

1. Resuscitation as required
2. Full neurological review to assess reasons for low GCS score
3. Bloods
4. Investigations: CT scan of the head (urgent), chest X-ray, urine for urinalysis, drug analysis and culture
5. Continuous reassessment and physiological monitoring as indicated

Additional information

Resuscitation

‣ Secure airway
‣ Oxygen: 100% initially, then ensure saturations are 94%–98%
‣ IV access
‣ Fluid resuscitate if BP <90 systolic

Full neurological examination

‣ Head and neck: trauma, neck stiffness (meningitis, subarachnoid haemorrhage), bruits
‣ Pupils: unilateral and fixed (requires urgent neurosurgical intervention); bilateral and fixed; pinpoint pupils; midpoint pupils
‣ Fundi – papilloedema
‣ Eye movements – conjugate lateral deviation of the eyes

Glasgow Coma Scale (minimum score 3, maximum score 15)

Best motor response		Best verbal response		Eyes open	
Obeys commands	6	Orientated	5	Spontaneously	4
Localises pain	5	Confused	4	Verbal command	3
Withdraws from pain	4	Inappropriate words	3	Pain	2
Abnormal flexion	3	Incomprehensible sounds	2	No response	1
Abnormal extension	2	No vocalisations	1		
No movement	1				

Blood tests

➲ Blood glucose (capillary)

➲ Arterial blood gas

➲ Venous: FBC, U&E, LFTs, Ca^{2+}, TFT, glucose, cortisol, ethanol/toxic screen, CK, Troponin I

➲ Blood cultures if temperature ≥38.0°C

Investigations

➲ 'Urgent' CT of the head as soon as possible, but certainly within 24 hours

➲ Lumbar puncture is required if mass lesion is excluded on CT and no signs of raised intracranial pressure

Monitoring

➲ Consider ITU or anaesthetic input if GCS score remains <8

Sepsis[20]

1. Administer high-flow oxygen
2. Blood cultures
3. IV antibiotics
4. Start IV fluid resuscitation
5. Check haemoglobin and lactate levels
6. Monitor accurate hourly urine output

Additional information

Systemic Inflammatory Response Syndrome criteria:

- ➲ Temperature <36.0°C or >38.3°C
- ➲ HR >90
- ➲ Respiration rate >20
- ➲ White cell count <4 or >12

Sepsis = Systemic Inflammatory Response Syndrome + identified infection
Severe sepsis = Sepsis + end organ damage

Oxygen

- ➲ Administer via a face mask and reservoir at 15 L/minute
  - Consider alternatives if patient has COPD (ensure saturations are between 88%–92%)

Antibiotics

- ➲ Prescribe antibiotics as per local policy
  - Discuss case with microbiologist if required

Fluid resuscitation

- ➲ Use Hartmann's solution

Blood tests

- ➲ Take a full set of laboratory bloods: FBC, U&E, LFTs, clotting

Urine output

- ➲ Consider catheterisation
- ➲ Urinalysis and send to the laboratory for MC&S

Disseminated intravascular coagulation

1. Resuscitation as required
2. Bloods
3. Correction of coagulopathy
4. Discuss with haematologist
5. Continuous reassessment and physiological monitoring as indicated

Additional information

Resuscitation

➲ Oxygen: ensure saturations are 94%–98%; if COPD, 88%–92%
➲ IV access
➲ Fluid resuscitate if BP <90 systolic

Blood tests

➲ Arterial blood gas as indicated
➲ Venous: FBC, U&E, clotting, X-match, D-dimer, fibrinogen

Correction of coagulopathy

➲ Fresh frozen plasma 15 mg/kg
➲ Platelets if <50 × 10⁹/L
➲ Blood transfusion if required
➲ Consider activated protein C if severe sepsis or multi organ failure

Monitoring

➲ Catheterise and monitor hourly output
➲ Consider ITU or anaesthetic input if patient deteriorating

Anaphylaxis[21]

1. Resuscitation as required
2. Administer adrenaline, hydrocortisone and chlorpheniramine
3. Bloods
4. Consider nebulised drugs
5. Continuous reassessment and physiological monitoring as indicated
6. Admit or discharge as appropriate

Additional information

Resuscitation

- Secure airway if indicated
- Oxygen: sit up with 100% initially
- Establish cause and stop further contact
- IV access
- Fluid resuscitate if BP <90 systolic
- Lie flat with feet raised if hypotensive

Dosages

- 500 mcg 1:1000 adrenaline IM
- Repeat every 5 minutes according to the patient's response
- Hydrocortisone 200 mg IV
- Chlorpheniramine 10 mg IV

Blood tests

- Arterial blood gas
- Venous: FBC, U&E; mast cell tryptase as soon as possible after emergency treatment has started, and a second blood sample no later than 4 hours after initial symptoms started

Nebulised drugs

- Salbutamol 5 mg
- Adrenaline 1:1000 solution, 5 mL (5 mg)

Monitoring

- Always consider ITU or anaesthetic input

Discharge

The following assistance should be offered by an appropriately trained healthcare professional before discharge.

➲ Information about anaphylaxis: signs and symptoms of an anaphylactic reaction; the risk of a biphasic reaction; what to do if an anaphylactic reaction occurs (use the adrenaline injector and call emergency services); the need for referral to a specialist allergy service and the referral process; patient support groups

➲ A demonstration of the correct use of the adrenaline injector and when to use it

➲ Advice about how to avoid the suspected trigger (if known)

Hypothermia

1. Resuscitation as required
2. Investigate and treat cause
3. Bloods
4. Investigations: chest X-ray, ECG
5. Continuous reassessment and physiological monitoring as indicated

Additional information

Resuscitation

⮞ Oxygen: ensure saturations are 94%–98%; if COPD, 88%–92%
⮞ IV access
⮞ Fluid resuscitate if BP <90 systolic
⮞ Attach cardiac monitoring

Investigate and treat cause of hypothermia

Investigation of hypothermia:
⮞ consider infection and treat appropriately

Treatment of hypothermia:
⮞ use warmed (37.0°C) IV fluids
⮞ passive external warming if temperature >32.0°C
⮞ active external warming if temperature 28.0°C–32.0°C
⮞ active internal warming if temperature <28.0°C
⮞ warm slowly – aim for 0.5°C per hour

Blood tests

⮞ Arterial blood gas
⮞ Venous: FBC, U&E, TFT, glucose
⮞ Blood cultures

Monitoring

⮞ Consider ITU or anaesthetic input if patient deteriorating

References

1. National Institute for Health and Clinical Excellence. *Chest Pain of Recent Onset: NICE clinical guideline 95*. London: NICE; 2010. www.nice.org.uk/CG95
2. Deakin CD, Nolan JP, Soar J, *et al*. European Resuscitation Council Guidelines for Resuscitation 2010: Section 4. Adult advanced life support. *Resuscitation*. 2010; **81**(10): 1305–52.
3. Scottish Intercollegiate Guidelines Network. *British Guideline on the Management of Asthma: a national clinical guideline 101*. Edinburgh: SIGN; 2009. www.sign. ac.uk/pdf/sign101.pdf
4. Lim WS, Baudouin SV, George RC, *et al*. Pneumonia Guidelines Committee of the BTS Standards of Care Committee. BTS guidelines for the management of community acquired pneumonia in adults: update 2009. *Thorax*. 2009; **64**(Suppl. 3): iii1–55.
5. O'Driscoll BR, Howard LS, Davison AG; British Thoracic Society. BTS guideline for emergency oxygen use in adult patients. *Thorax*. 2008; **63**(Suppl. 6): vi1–68.
6. Henry M, Arnold T, Harvey J; Pleural Diseases Group, Standards of Care Committee, British Thoracic Society. BTS guidelines for the management of spontaneous pneumothorax. *Thorax*. 2003; **58**(Suppl. 2): ii39–52.
7. National Institute for Health and Clinical Excellence. *Venous Thromboembolic Diseases: NICE clinical guideline 144*. London: NICE; 2012. www.nice.org.uk/ CG144
8. National Institute for Health and Clinical Excellence. *Chronic Obstructive Pulmonary Disease: NICE clinical guideline 101*. London: NICE; 2010. www.nice.org.uk/CG101
9. British Thoracic Society Standards of Care Committee. NIPPV non-invasive ventilation in acute respiratory failure. *Thorax*. 2002; **57**(3): 192–211.
10. National Institute for Health and Clinical Excellence. *Acute Upper GI Bleeding: NICE clinical guideline 141*. London: NICE; 2012. www.nice.org.uk/CG141
11. Scottish Intercollegiate Guidelines Network. *Diagnosis and Management of Headache in Adults: SIGN guideline 107*. Edinburgh: SIGN; 2008. www.sign.ac.uk/ pdf/sign107.pdf
12. National Institute for Health and Clinical Excellence. *Headaches: NICE clinical guideline 150*. London: NICE; 2012. www.nice.org.uk/CG150
13. National Institute for Health and Clinical Excellence. *The Epilepsies: NICE clinical guideline 137*. London: NICE; 2012. www.nice.org.uk/CG137
14. National Institute for Health and Clinical Excellence. *Stroke: NICE clinical guideline 68*. London: NICE; 2008. www.nice.org.uk/CG68
15. Bederson JB, Connolly ES Jr, Batjer HH, *et al*. American Heart Association. Guidelines for the management of aneurysmal subarachnoid hemorrhage. *Stroke*. 2009; **40**(3): 994–1025.
16. Scottish Intercollegiate Guidelines Network. *Management of Suspected Bacterial Urinary Tract Infection in Adults: SIGN guideline 88*. Edinburgh: SIGN; 2012. www. sign.ac.uk/pdf/sign88.pdf
17. National Institute for Health and Clinical Excellence. *Type 1 Diabetes: NICE clinical guideline 15*. London: NICE; 2004. www.nice.org.uk/CG15
18. Outterside K, Sankar S, Syed A. *Hyperosmolar Hyperglycaemic Non-Ketotic*

Coma (HONK). Available at: http://acutemed.co.uk/diseases/Hyperosmolar +Hyperglycaemic+Non-Ketotic+Coma+(HONK)# (accessed 1 August 2014).

19. Brackenridge A, Wallbank H, Lawrenson RA, *et al.* Emergency management of diabetes and hypoglycaemia. *Emerg Med J.* 2006; **23**(3): 183–5.

20. survivesepsis.org

21. National Institute for Health and Clinical Excellence. *Anaphylaxis: NICE clinical guideline 134.* London: NICE; 2011. www.nice.org.uk/CG134

3

SURGICAL EMERGENCIES

Septic joint

1. Resuscitation as required
2. Splint joint and request an urgent orthopaedic opinion
3. Bloods
4. Investigations: joint X-ray, joint aspiration
5. Analgesia
6. Antibiotics

Additional information

Resuscitation

- Oxygen: ensure saturations are 94%–98%; if COPD, 88%–92%
- IV access
- Fluid resuscitate if BP <90 systolic
- IV fluids – normal maintenance
- NBM

Blood tests

- Venous: FBC, U&E, CRP, ESR, urate
- Blood cultures

Analgesia

- Paracetamol 1 g ± codeine 60 mg, or
- Titrate morphine by slow IV administration

Antibiotics

- Flucloxacillin 2 g qds IV and benzylpenicillin 2.4 g qds IV
- Antibiotic administration is dependent on local policy

Acute lower back pain (atraumatic)[1]

1. Full history and examination to differentiate between causes
2. Bloods
3. Investigations: urinalysis
4. Analgesia
5. Consider urgent surgical referral if:
   - red flag signs present
   - cauda equina syndrome considered
6. Discharge simple back pain to GP with adequate analgesia

Additional information
Blood tests
⮕ Venous: FBC, U&E, CRP, prostate-specific antigen (if male and over 55)

Investigations
⮕ Spinal X-ray is not recommended
⮕ Consider MRI when any of the following diagnoses are suspected:
   - spinal malignancy, infection, fracture, cauda equina syndrome, ankylosing spondylitis or another inflammatory disorder

Analgesia
⮕ Paracetamol 1 g ± ibuprofen 200 or 400 mg, or
⮕ Titrate morphine by slow IV administration

Red flag signs
⮕ Lower limb weakness
⮕ Altered perineal sensation
⮕ Altered perianal sensation
⮕ Sphincter disturbance

Spinal cord compression[1]

1. Full history and examination
2. Analgesia
3. Bloods
4. Investigations: chest X-ray, urgent MRI spine
5. Urgent neurosurgical referral if cauda equina syndrome considered

Additional information

Analgesia
➲ Paracetamol 1 g ± ibuprofen 200 or 400 mg, or
➲ Titrate morphine by slow IV administration

Blood tests
➲ Venous: FBC, U&E, CRP, B_{12}, folate

Investigations
➲ MRI scan is considered when any of the following diagnoses are suspected:
  • spinal malignancy, infection, fracture, cauda equina syndrome, ankylosing spondylitis or another inflammatory disorder
➲ Consider spinal X-ray if urgent MRI unavailable

Red flag signs
➲ Lower limb weakness
➲ Altered perineal sensation
➲ Altered perianal sensation
➲ Sphincter disturbance

Testicular torsion

1. Senior review immediately
2. Analgesia
3. Bloods
4. Investigations: consider a Doppler scan, urinalysis
5. Urgent surgical opinion

Additional information

Immediate senior review

➲ Ensure patient is NBM and has IV access while waiting for senior review

Analgesia

➲ Paracetamol 1 g ± codeine 60 mg, or
➲ Titrate morphine by slow IV administration

Blood tests

➲ Venous: FBC, U&E, CRP

Investigations

➲ A Doppler scan is often useful to assess blood supply but should not delay referral

Aortic dissection

1. Resuscitation as required
2. Analgesia
3. Bloods
4. Investigations: chest X-ray, CT of the thorax and abdomen, echocardiogram, ECG
5. Urgent cardiothoracic referral
6. Continuous reassessment and physiological monitoring as indicated

Additional information

Resuscitation

➲ Oxygen 100% initially
➲ IV access
➲ IV fluid resuscitation as indicated
➲ NBM

Analgesia

➲ Paracetamol 1 g ± codeine 60 mg, or
➲ Titrate morphine by slow IV administration

Blood tests

➲ Venous: FBC, U&E, LFTs, clotting, glucose
➲ X-match for 6 units

Monitoring

➲ Maintain systolic BP <100 mmHg:
  • discuss with cardiology or cardiothoracic surgeons reference management of BP
➲ Catheterise and monitor hourly output
➲ Consider ITU or anaesthetic input if patient deteriorating

Limb ischaemia

1. Analgesia
2. Bloods
3. Investigations: arteriography, chest X-ray, Doppler to assess pulses, ECG, urinalysis (myoglobin)
4. Urgent surgical opinion
5. Continuous reassessment for changes in limb ischaemia

Additional information

Analgesia

⊃ Paracetamol 1 g ± codeine 60 mg, or
⊃ Titrate morphine by slow IV administration

Blood tests

⊃ Venous: FBC, U&E, LFTs, CRP, ESR, CK, clotting, lipids, glucose
⊃ Group and save

Indicators of limb ischaemia

⊃ Pale
⊃ Pulseless
⊃ Painful
⊃ Paralysis
⊃ Paraesthetic
⊃ Perishing cold
⊃ Fixed mottling implies irreversibility

Appendicitis

1. Resuscitation as required
2. Follow sepsis pathway if indicated
3. Analgesia
4. Bloods
5. Investigations: CT or USS if considering appendix mass, pregnancy test in women of childbearing age, urinalysis
6. Surgical opinion

Additional information

Resuscitation

➲ Oxygen: ensure saturations are 94%–98%; if COPD, 88%–92%
➲ IV access
➲ Fluid resuscitate if BP <90 systolic
➲ Fluids depending on dehydration status + normal maintenance
➲ NBM

Analgesia

➲ Paracetamol 1 g ± codeine 60 mg, or
➲ Titrate morphine by slow IV administration

Blood tests

➲ Venous: FBC, U&E, LFTs, CRP, ESR
➲ Blood cultures if temperature ≥38°C
➲ Group and save

Acute pancreatitis[2]

1. Resuscitation as required
2. Identify future potential complications using the Glasgow Criteria
3. Analgesia
4. Bloods
5. Investigations: pregnancy test in women of childbearing age, urinalysis
6. Surgical opinion for further management and investigations

Additional information

Resuscitation

- Oxygen: ensure saturations are 94%–98%; if COPD, 88%–92%
- IV access
- Fluid resuscitate if BP <90 systolic
- Fluids depending on dehydration status + normal maintenance
- NBM
- NG tube

Glasgow criteria

P_aO_2	<8 kPa
Age	>55 years
Neutrophils	White cell count >15 ≥ 10^9/L
Calcium	<2 mmol/L
Renal function	Urea >16 mmol/L
Enzymes	LDH >600 iu/L; AST >200 iu/L
Albumin	<32 g/L (serum)
Sugar	Blood glucose >10 mmol/L

A score >3 predicts complications.

Analgesia

- Titrate morphine by slow IV administration, or
- Pethidine 75 mg qds IM

Blood tests
- ⊃ Arterial blood gas
- ⊃ Venous: FBC, U&E, LFTs, CRP, Ca²⁺, amylase, lipase, glucose, clotting
- ⊃ Blood cultures if temperature ≥38.0°C
- ⊃ Group and save

While waiting for a surgical opinion
- ⊃ Catheterise and monitor hourly output
- ⊃ Consider ITU or anaesthetic input if patient deteriorating

Acute cholecystitis

1. Resuscitation as required
2. Analgesia
3. Bloods
4. Investigations: erect chest X-ray, pregnancy test in women of childbearing age, urinalysis, USS of the abdomen
5. Consider antibiotics and a surgical opinion

Additional information

Resuscitation

⮞ Oxygen: ensure saturations are 94%–98%; if COPD, 88%–92%
⮞ Follow sepsis pathway if indicated
⮞ IV access
⮞ Fluid resuscitate if BP <90 systolic
⮞ Fluids depending on dehydration status + normal maintenance
⮞ NG tube if vomiting
⮞ NBM

Analgesia

⮞ Titrate morphine by slow IV administration, or
⮞ Pethidine 75 mg qds IM

Blood tests

⮞ Venous: FBC, U&E, LFTs, CRP, amylase, clotting
⮞ Blood cultures if temperature ≥38.0°C
⮞ Group and save

Investigations

⮞ An erect chest X-ray is required to exclude a perforation

Antibiotic regimen

⮞ Cefuroxime 1.5 g tds IV and metronidazole 500 mg tds IV
⮞ Antibiotic administration is dependent on local policy

Renal colic[3]

1. Resuscitation as required
2. Analgesia
3. Bloods
4. Investigations: KUB X-ray or CTKUB depending on local policy, pregnancy test in females of childbearing age, urinalysis and midstream specimen of urine, USS or Doppler in patients with renal impairment or pregnancy
5. Antibiotics if infection present
6. Consider surgical referral:
   - if discharged, inform patient to arrange appointment with their GP

Additional information

Resuscitation

➲ Oxygen: ensure saturations are 94%–98%; if COPD, 88%–92%
➲ Follow sepsis pathway if indicated
➲ Rule out abdominal aortic aneurysm

Analgesia

➲ Diclofenac 75–150 mg daily PO in two to three divided doses, or
➲ Titrate morphine by slow IV administration, or
➲ Pethidine 75 mg qds IM

Blood tests

➲ Venous: FBC, U&E, CRP, Ca^{2+}, PO_4^{3-}, glucose, clotting, urate
➲ Blood cultures if temperature ≥38.0°C
➲ Group and save

Antibiotic regimen

➲ Cefuroxime 1.5 g tds IV and metronidazole 500 mg tds IV
➲ Antibiotics are dependent on local policy

Contact surgeons for admission in patients

➲ Whose pain cannot be resolved
➲ Who have signs of sepsis
➲ Who have new-onset renal impairment
➲ Whose investigations confirm obstruction or hydronephrosis
➲ Or other locally agreed criteria

Gastrointestinal haemorrhage (lower)[4]

1. Resuscitation as required
2. Bloods
3. Investigations: ECG; consider referral for localisation of bleeding point
4. Correct any clotting abnormalities
5. Continuous reassessment and physiological monitoring
6. Urgent surgical opinion if patient is haemodynamically unstable

Additional information

Resuscitation

- Oxygen: ensure saturations are 94%–98%; if COPD, 88%–92%
- IV access
- Fluid resuscitate if BP <90 systolic
- NG tube if vomiting
- NBM
- Place patient flat with feet raised if hypotensive or lateral position if vomiting

Blood tests

- Arterial blood gas as indicated
- Venous: FBC, U&E, LFTs, clotting, glucose
- X-match for 6 units

Investigations

Consider referring for the following investigations to localise the bleeding point:

- CT scan, CT angiography or digital subtraction angiography

Correcting clotting abnormalities

- Vitamin K, clotting factors, or fresh frozen plasma in accordance with local policy

Monitoring

- Monitor hourly output (consider catheterisation)
- Consider CVP monitoring
- Consider ITU or anaesthetic input if patient deteriorating

Intestinal obstruction

1. Resuscitation as required
2. Analgesia
3. Bloods
4. Investigations: abdominal X-ray, pregnancy test in women of childbearing age, urinalysis
5. Continuous reassessment and physiological monitoring
6. Urgent surgical opinion

Additional information

Resuscitation

- Oxygen: ensure saturations are 94%–98%; if COPD, 88%–92%
- IV access
- Fluid resuscitate if BP <90 systolic
- Fluids depending on dehydration status + normal maintenance
- NG tube if vomiting
- NBM
- Follow sepsis pathway if indicated
- Consider ITU or anaesthetic input if patient deteriorating

Analgesia

- Paracetamol 1 g ± codeine 60 mg, or
- Titrate morphine by slow IV administration

Blood tests

- Arterial blood gas as indicated
- Venous: FBC, U&E, LFTs, CRP, glucose, clotting
- Blood cultures if temperature ≥38.0°C
- Group and save

Acute urinary retention

1. Resuscitation as required
2. Analgesia
3. Urethral catheterisation
4. Bloods
5. Investigations: renal ultrasound in renal impairment, urinalysis and midstream specimen of urine
6. Urology or surgical opinion

Additional information

Resuscitation
- Oxygen: ensure saturations are 94%–98%; if COPD, 88%–92%
- IV access
- Fluid resuscitate if BP <90 systolic
- Fluids depending on dehydration status + normal maintenance
- Follow sepsis pathway if indicated

Analgesia
- Paracetamol 1 g + codeine 60 mg, or
- Titrate morphine by slow IV administration

Catheterisation
- Consider suprapubic catheter if urethral catheterisation impossible or contraindicated

Blood tests
- Arterial blood gas as indicated
- Venous: FBC, U&E, LFTs, CRP, amylase, glucose, clotting, prostate-specific antigen
- Blood cultures if temperature ≥38.0°C
- Group and save

Shock

1. Resuscitation as required
2. Bloods
3. Commence fluid resuscitation using crystalloid (1 L STAT)
4. Identify underlying cause and commence directed therapy
5. Continuous reassessment and physiological monitoring

Additional information

Classification of shock

- Hypovolaemic (↑HR, ↓BP, cool peripheries, fluid or blood loss, ↓urine output)
- Septic or inflammatory (↑HR, ↓BP, warm peripheries, source or suspicion of infection)
- Cardiogenic (underlying cardiac disease, signs of heart failure)
- Neurogenic (recent injury or trauma, focal neurological signs)

Resuscitation

- Secure airway as indicated
- Oxygen: sit up with 100% initially, then ensure saturations are 94%–98%
- IV access
- If no output detected, commence cardiopulmonary resuscitation and call the resuscitation team

Blood tests

- Arterial blood gas as indicated
- Venous bloods: FBC, U&E, lactate, coagulation screen, glucose, LFTs, CRP
- Blood cultures if indicated
- X-match

Fluid administration

- Monitor physiological response (BP, HR, capillary refill)
- Use response to guide to further fluid resuscitation

Monitoring

- Catheterise and monitor hourly output
- Consider CVP monitoring
- Consider ITU or anaesthetic input

References

1. National Institute for Health and Clinical Excellence. *Low back pain: NICE guideline 88*. London: NICE; 2009. www.nice.org.uk/CG88
2. Working Party of the British Society of Gastroenterology; Association of Surgeons of Great Britain and Ireland; Pancreatic Society of Great Britain and Ireland; Association of Upper GI Surgeons of Great Britain and Ireland. UK guidelines for the management of acute pancreatitis. *Gut.* 2005; **54**(Suppl. 3): iii1–9.
3. British Association of Urological Surgeons. *Guidelines for Acute Management of First Presentation of Renal/Ureteric Lithiasis*. London: BAUS; 2008; reviewed 2012. Available at: www.baus.org.uk/Resources/BAUS/Documents/PDF%20 Documents/Sections/Endourology/Revised%20Acute%20Stone%20Mgt%20 Guidelines.pdf (accessed 1 October 2012).
4. Scottish Intercollegiate Guidelines Network. *Management of Acute Upper and Lower Gastrointestinal Bleeding: SIGN guideline 105.* Edinburgh: SIGN; 2008. www.sign.ac.uk/pdf/sign105.pdf

4

WOMEN AND CHILDREN'S HEALTH

Women

Ectopic pregnancy[1,2]

1. Resuscitate as required
2. Confirm pregnancy
3. Bloods
4. Consider early surgical referral
5. Consider anti-D immunoglobulin

Additional information

Resuscitation

- ➲ Oxygen: ensure saturations are 94%–98%; if COPD, 88%–92%
- ➲ IV access
- ➲ Fluid resuscitate if BP <90 systolic
- ➲ Fluids depending on dehydration status + normal maintenance
- ➲ Follow sepsis pathway if indicated

Confirm pregnancy

- ➲ Urine beta hCG level
- ➲ Determine gestation (history or patient's records)

Blood tests

- ➲ Venous: FBC, U&E, clotting, rhesus and antibody status
- ➲ X-match

Surgical referral

- ➲ If suspected ruptured ectopic, seek early specialist (gynaecological and anaesthetic) input and inform theatres.

Anti-D immunoglobulin

- ➲ Non-sensitised women who are rhesus negative with a confirmed or suspected ectopic pregnancy should receive anti-D immunoglobulin.

Vaginal bleeding in pregnancy[2,3]

1. Resuscitate as required
2. Check pregnancy status
3. Bloods
4. Consider anti-D immunoglobulin
5. Further management

If bleeding continues:
➲ referral to gynaecology for full assessment
➲ send any tissue passed to histology.

*If bleeding is minimal (less than normal period) and patient haemody-
namically stable:*
➲ consider discharge with early gynaecology follow-up or USS, dependent
  on local provision –
  ● ensure case is discussed with on-call gynaecologist prior to discharge
  ● send any tissue passed to histology.

Additional information

Resuscitation
➲ Oxygen: ensure saturations are 94%–98%; if COPD, 88%–92%
➲ IV access
➲ Fluid resuscitate if BP <90 systolic
➲ Fluids depending on dehydration status + normal maintenance
➲ Follow sepsis pathway if indicated

Confirm pregnancy
➲ Urine beta hCG level (if negative send serum beta hCG)
➲ Determine gestation (history or patient's records)

Blood tests
➲ Venous: FBC, U&E, rhesus and antibody status
➲ Group and save or X-match – depending on extent of bleed

Anti D-immunoglobulin: administration

➲ Non-sensitised rhesus (Rh) negative women should receive anti-D immunoglobulin in the following situations: ectopic pregnancy, all miscarriages over 12 weeks of gestation (including threatened) and all miscarriages where the uterus is evacuated (whether medically or surgically).

➲ Anti-D immunoglobulin should only be given for threatened miscarriage under 12 weeks' gestation when bleeding is heavy or associated with pain. It is not required for cases of complete miscarriage under 12 weeks of gestation when there has been no formal intervention to evacuate the uterus.

Children

Croup

1. Calculate a croup score
2. Avoid distressing the child and allow parents to look after the child

Mild to moderate croup (croup score 1–4)

3. Humidified oxygen if hypoxia present
4. Steroids
5. Repeat croup score at 2 hours

Severe croup (croup score >5)

3. Humidified oxygen if hypoxia present
4. Nebulised adrenaline
5. Improvement may be rapid but rebound effect can occur up to 2 hours post treatment
6. Steroids

Additional information

Croup score

Stridor	Score
None	0
On crying or exertion	1
At rest	2
Biphasic	3

Recessions	Score
None	0
On crying or exertion	1
At rest	2
Severe	3

Mild to moderate croup (croup score 1–4)

Steroids

➲ Oral dexamethasone 0.15 mg/kg

Repeat croup score at 2 hours

➲ If child improved and croup score 0, discharge with advice
➲ If improved but croup score >0, discuss with senior prior to discharge
➲ If patient no better or deteriorating, refer to paediatrics

Severe croup (croup score >5)

Humidified oxygen
➲ Hypoxia <94%

Nebulised adrenaline
➲ Oxygen-driven nebulised adrenaline 1:1000 0.4 mL/kg (maximum 5 mL)

Consider specialist support
➲ Seek early specialist input if no improvement or rebound effect (anaesthetics; paediatrics; ear, nose and throat)

Steroids
➲ Oral dexamethasone 0.15 mg/kg if tolerated

Bronchiolitis[4]

1. Obtain baseline observations and oxygen saturations
2. Assess for signs of respiratory distress
3. Allow parents to look after the child to avoid distress
4. Avoid routine use of bronchodilators or steroids
5. Continuous reassessment and monitoring
6. Consider referral to paediatrics

Additional information

Oxygen requirements

- ➲ 100% oxygen via face mask if signs of hypoxia or oxygen saturations <92%

Clinical signs of respiratory distress

- ➲ Recessions (intercostal, subcostal)
- ➲ Chest crackles
- ➲ Tracheal tug
- ➲ Wheeze
- ➲ Nasal flaring
- ➲ Head bobbing

Referral to paediatric specialist if any of the following are present

- ➲ Hypoxia, oxygen saturations ≤92%
- ➲ Witnessed or suspected apnoea
- ➲ Respiratory rate >70 breaths a minute
- ➲ Presence of nasal flaring or grunting
- ➲ Severe chest wall recession
- ➲ Cyanosis
- ➲ <50% normal fluid input in last 24 hours
- ➲ Lethargy
- ➲ Uncertainty regarding diagnosis
- ➲ Significant co-morbidities
- ➲ <3 months old
- ➲ Born at <35/40 weeks' gestation
- ➲ Consider parental ability to cope

Asthma: age 2–5 years[5]

1. Assess asthma severity

Moderate

2. Administer inhaler
3. Steroids
4. Reassess in 1 hour
5. Consider discharge

Severe

2. Oxygen
3. Administer inhaler or nebuliser
4. Steroids
5. Continuous reassessment and physiological monitoring
6. Inform senior and contact paediatric intensive care unit (PICU) if poor response to treatment

Life-threatening

2. Oxygen
3. Nebulisers
4. Steroids
5. Continuous reassessment and physiological monitoring
6. Inform senior and contact PICU if poor response to treatment

Additional information

Asthma severity

Moderate

- SpO_2 ≥92%
- No clinical features of severe asthma

Severe

- SpO_2 <92%
- Use of accessory neck muscles
- Respirations >40 breaths per minute
- Pulse >140 beats per minute
- Too breathless to talk or feed

Life-threatening (severe + one of the following)

- Agitation
- Silent chest
- Cyanosis
- Poor respiratory effort
- Altered consciousness

Moderate

Inhalers

- Salbutamol 2–10 puffs via spacer ± face mask, repeat every 2 minutes up to 10 puffs

Steroid therapy

- Soluble oral prednisolone 20 mg

Discharge plan

- Continue beta2-agonist every 4 hours as required
- Consider prednisolone 20 mg for 3 days
- Advise to contact GP if not controlled
- Provide a written asthma action plan
- Review regular treatment
- Check inhaler treatment
- Arrange GP follow-up

Severe

Oxygen

- Oxygen via face mask or nasal prongs to achieve 94%–98% saturations

Inhaler or nebulisers

- Salbutamol inhaler, 10 puffs via spacer ± face mask, or
- Salbutamol nebuliser 2.5 mg and ipratropium bromide nebuliser 250 mcg

Repeat every 20–30 minutes according to response.

Steroids

- Oral prednisolone 20 mg or IV hydrocortisone 4 mg/kg if vomiting

Life-threatening

Oxygen

➲ Oxygen via face mask or nasal prongs to achieve 94%–98% saturations

Nebulisers

➲ Salbutamol 2.5 mg and ipratropium bromide 250 mcg

Repeat every 20–30 minutes.

Steroids

➲ Oral prednisolone 20 mg or IV hydrocortisone 4 mg/kg if vomiting

Asthma: age >5 years[5]

1. Assess asthma severity

Moderate

2. Administer inhaler
3. Steroids
4. Reassess in 1 hour
5. Consider discharge

Severe

2. Oxygen
3. Administer inhaler or nebuliser
4. Steroids
5. Continuous reassessment and physiological monitoring
6. Inform senior and contact PICU if poor response to treatment

Life-threatening

2. Oxygen
3. Nebulisers
4. Steroids
5. Continuous reassessment and physiological monitoring
6. Inform senior and contact PICU if poor response to treatment

Additional information

Asthma severity

Moderate

➲ SpO_2 ≥92%
➲ PEFR ≥50% of best or predicted
➲ No clinical features of severe asthma

Severe

➲ SpO_2 <92%
➲ PEFR <33% – 50% of best or predicted
➲ Respiratory rate ≥30 breaths per minute
➲ Pulse >125 beats per minute
➲ Use of accessory neck muscles

Life-threatening (severe + one of the following)
- PEFR <33% best or predicted
- Cyanosis
- Poor respiratory effort
- Silent chest
- Altered consciousness

Moderate
Inhalers
- Salbutamol 2–10 puffs via spacer ± face mask, repeat every 2 minutes up to 10 puffs

Steroid therapy
- Oral prednisolone 30–40 mg

Discharge plan
- Continue beta2-agonist every 4 hours as required
- Consider prednisolone 20 mg for 3 days
- Advise to contact GP if not controlled
- Provide a written asthma action plan
- Review regular treatment
- Check inhaler treatment
- Arrange GP follow-up

Severe
Oxygen
- Oxygen via face mask or nasal prongs to achieve 94%–98% saturations

Inhaler/nebulisers
- Salbutamol inhaler 10 puffs via spacer ± face mask, or
- Salbutamol nebuliser 2.5–5 mg

Repeat every 20–30 minutes according to response.
- If poor response, add ipratropium bromide nebuliser 250 mcg.

Repeat every 20–30 minutes according to response.

Steroids

⊃ Oral prednisolone 30–40 mg or IV hydrocortisone 4 mg/kg if vomiting

Life-threatening

Oxygen

⊃ Oxygen via face mask or nasal prongs to achieve 94%–98% saturations

Nebulisers

⊃ Salbutamol nebuliser 5 mg and ipratropium bromide nebuliser 250 mcg

Repeat every 20–30 minutes.

Steroids

⊃ Oral prednisolone 30–40 mg or IV hydrocortisone 4 mg/kg if vomiting

Febrile child[6]

1. Identify underlying cause through history and examination
2. Assessment of serious illness
3. Antipyretics if the child is distressed
4. Consider bloods if child is to be admitted
5. Investigations (tailored to severity of illness)

Additional information
Assessment of serious illness

➲ Assess for compromise of the airway, breathing, circulation or a decreased level of consciousness. Transfer to the resuscitation room if any present.
➲ If signs or symptoms of severe infection/sepsis or meningitis, then obtain early senior assistance and begin empirical antibiotic treatment based on local policy.
➲ The following groups should be considered as being in a high-risk group for serious illness:
   ● children younger than 3 months with a temperature of 38°C or higher
   ● children aged 3–6 months with a temperature of 39°C or higher.

Assess as per the traffic light system
Children with *red* features (but no immediately life-threatening illness):
➲ refer urgently to the care of a paediatric specialist.

Children with *amber* features:
➲ if no diagnosis has been reached consider referral to a paediatric specialist for further assessment.

Children with *green* features (and none of the amber or red features):
➲ can be managed at home with appropriate advice for parents and carers, including advice on when to seek further attention from the healthcare services as per local policy.

Traffic light system

	Green – low risk	Amber – intermediate risk	Red – high risk
Colour	Normal colour of skin, lips and tongue	Pallor reported by parent or carer	Pale, mottled, ashen or blue
Activity	Responds normally to social cues Content/smiles Stays awake or awakens quickly Strong normal cry or not crying	Not responding normally to social cues Wakes only with prolonged stimulation Decreased activity No smile	No response to social cues Appears ill to a healthcare professional Unable to rouse or, if roused, does not stay awake Weak, high-pitched or continuous cry
Respiratory		Nasal flaring Tachypnoea: • RR >50 breaths per minute, aged 6–12 months • RR >40 breaths per minute, aged >12 months • Oxygen saturation –95% in air • Crackles	Grunting Tachypnoea: • RR >60 breaths a minute • moderate or severe chest in-drawing
Hydration	Normal skin and eyes Moist mucous membranes	Dry mucous membrane Poor feeding in infants CRT × 3 seconds Reduced urine output	Reduced skin turgor
Other	**None** of the amber or red symptoms or signs	Fever for ×5 days	Age 0–3 months, temperature ≥38°C Age 3–6 months, temperature ≥39°C
		Swelling of a limb or joint Non-weight-bearing or not using an extremity	Non-blanching rash Bulging fontanelle Neck stiffness Status epilepticus Focal neurological signs Focal seizures

CRT, capillary refill time; RR, respiratory rate

Antipyretics

➲ Paracetamol and (or) ibuprofen as per local policy

Blood tests

➲ Venous: FBC, U&E, CRP
➲ Blood cultures

Investigations

➲ Chest X-ray
➲ Urinalysis and midstream specimen of urine
➲ Lumbar puncture

Apnoea

1. Resuscitate as required following Advanced Paediatric Life Support guidelines
2. Obtain details of event from history and confirm if an apnoeic episode has occurred
3. Identify any underlying cause or significant pathology
4. Further investigation should be based on clinical suspicion and the history
5. Admission to paediatrics in all infants (up to 1 year) who present with a first episode of apnoea

Additional information

Review of history

➲ Type of event and duration
➲ Any previous episodes?
➲ Requiring encouragement or stimulation to breathe
➲ Any change in colour?
➲ Changes in muscle tone (stiffness or limpness)

Status epilepticus

1. If actively fitting resuscitate following Advanced Paediatric Life Support principles
2. Check blood glucose
3. If seizure stops, seek early senior input for ongoing management
4. If seizure continues:
   - at 5 minutes –
     - › IV/IO lorazepam 0.1 mg/kg, or
     - › if no IV/IO access, midazolam buccal 0.5 mg/kg or diazepam per rectum 0.5 mg/kg
   - after another 10 minutes –
     - › IV/IO lorazepam 0.1 mg/kg
     - › call for senior help
   - After another 10 minutes –
     - › obtain senior, anaesthetist and PICU support as required
     - › phenytoin infusion IV/IO 20 mg/kg over 20 minutes
     - › or if already on phenytoin, phenobarbitone 20 mg/kg IV/IO over 5 minutes
5. If seizure does not stop, then prepare for a rapid sequence induction with thiopental

Additional information

Resuscitation

- ➲ Secure airway
- ➲ 100% oxygen via face mask

Blood glucose

- ➲ If <3 mmol/L (or you cannot obtain a blood glucose), administer 2 mL/kg of 10% glucose, followed by a 5 mL/kg/hour infusion of 10% glucose with 0.45% saline

Controlled seizure

- ➲ Assess child for underlying cause
- ➲ Reassessment and physiological monitoring

Identifying underlying cause

- ⇒ Blood gas
- ⇒ Venous bloods: FBC, U&E, LFTs, glucose, Ca^{2+}, Mg^{2+}, clotting screen
- ⇒ Blood cultures
- ⇒ Chest X-ray
- ⇒ Urinalysis and MC&S
- ⇒ Anticonvulsant levels as required
- ⇒ Lumbar puncture

Pulled elbow (subluxation of the radial head)

1. Review history
2. Reassurance to parents and child
3. Reduce elbow
4. Allow the child to settle and play post reduction
5. Home with advice

Additional information

Classic history

➲ Direct pull on the arm of a child aged <5 years followed by the child refusing to use the arm

How reduction can be achieved

➲ Flexing affected limb at elbow to 90°
➲ Full supination of elbow – a 'click' is sometime felt on relocation
➲ Alternatively, full pronation of the elbow may be used

Post reduction

➲ If the child begins to use the arm reduction has been achieved
➲ If the child does not begin to use the arm, seek senior advice regarding X-ray

Advice

➲ Avoid lifting or swinging child by the arms

References

1. Royal College of Obstetricians and Gynaecologists. *Tubal Pregnancy, Management: RCOG guideline No. 21*. London: RCOG; 2010. www.rcog.org.uk/files/rcog-corp/GTG21_230611.pdf
2. National Institute for Health and Clinical Excellence. *Ectopic Pregnancy and Miscarriage: NICE clinical guideline 154*. London: NICE; 2012. www.nice.org.uk/CG154
3. Royal College of Obstetricians and Gynaecologists. *The Management of Early Pregnancy Loss: green-top guideline No. 25*. London: RCOG; 2006. www.rcog.org.uk/files/rcog-corp/uploaded-files/GT25ManagementofEarlyPregnancyLoss2006.pdf
4. Scottish Intercollegiate Guidelines Network. *Bronchiolitis in Children: SIGN guideline 91*. Edinburgh: SIGN; 2006. www.sign.ac.uk/pdf/sign91.pdf
5. Scottish Intercollegiate Guidelines Network. *British Guideline on the Management of Asthma: SIGN Guideline 101*. Edinburgh: SIGN; Revised 2012. www.sign.ac.uk/pdf/sign101.pdf
6. National Institute for Health and Care Excellence. *Feverish Illness in Children: NICE clinical guideline 160*. London: NICE; 2013. www.nice.org.uk/CG160

Further reading

Advanced Life Support Group. *Advanced Paediatric Life Support*. 5th revised ed. Hoboken, NJ: John Wiley & Sons (Wiley-Blackwell); 2011.

5

ELDERLY CARE AND BEREAVEMENT

Frail elderly discharge

1. Ensure patient is medically fit for discharge
2. Asses mental state using 'Abbreviated Mental State' and capacity – compare with normal from collateral history, GP, past admission notes
3. Ensure patient can mobilise safely and appropriate aids are provided
4. Document any changes to medication and inform GP and carers
5. Follow up as indicated
6. Consider barriers to the patient's discharge

Additional information

Points to consider prior to discharge

➲ Lying and standing BP (postural drop)
➲ ECG (cardiac condition, arrhythmia)
➲ Urinalysis
➲ Chest X-ray, if clinically indicated (chest infection)

Follow up as indicated

➲ Inform GP
➲ Referral to specialist clinic (falls, TIA)
➲ Home assessment
➲ Restart care package

Barriers to a patient's discharge

➲ Evidence of self-neglect
➲ Increasing confusion late at night
➲ Patient lives alone
➲ Safeguarding issues

Bereavement care

1. Use the SPIKES strategy to prepare for breaking bad news
2. Introduce yourself and allow others present to do the same
3. Provide a clear and jargon-free explanation
4. Provide details of 'what happens next' as guided by local policy
5. Allow time for questions and provide contact details as appropriate
6. Arrange follow-up care

Additional information

SPIKES strategy for breaking bad news

Setting:

- set the scene by ensuring the privacy of your conversation
- select a quiet and private place in which to break the bad news
- greet your patients warmly, with a smile and make eye contact
- ensure there are no physical barriers between you and your patients

Perception:

- assess patients' perceptions of their illnesses by asking open-ended questions
- remember the vocabulary that the patient uses and repeat his or her choice of words when you break the news

Invitation:

- invitation to impart medical information should come from your patients
- the vast majority of your patients will want to know the details of their illness, but to respect those who don't, be sure to ask their preference

Knowledge:

- knowledge should be shared with your patients by replicating their vocabulary
- give your patients small chunks of information, making sure that they understand the content after each chunk

Empathising and Exploring:

➲ empathic and exploratory responses should be used when responding to your patients' emotions on hearing bad news

➲ validate their feelings

Details

➲ Provide details and written information if possible on local bereavement services and counselling

6

MENTAL HEALTH EMERGENCIES

Deliberate self-harm[1]

1. Full assessment of suicide risk, e.g. the SADPERSONS scale
2. Physical and mental state examination
3. Contact mental health services as per local policy
4. Disposal is dependent on assessment and local policy
5. Provide any literature available on community groups and support systems

Additional information

SADPERSONS scale	Score
Sex (male)	1
Age (<19 and >45)	1
Depression or hopelessness	2
Previous attempts or psychiatric care	1
Excessive alcohol or drug use	1
Rational thinking loss (psychiatric or organic illness)	2
Separated, widowed or divorced	1
Organised or serious attempt	2
No social support	1
State future intent	2

➲ Score <6: may be safe for discharge (consider circumstances)
➲ Score 6–8: requires psychiatric review
➲ Score >8: candidate for hospital admission with psychiatric review

Poisoning

1. Resuscitation as required
2. History of events and assessment of substances taken or suicidal intent
3. Bloods
4. Continuous reassessment and physiological monitoring
5. Provide any literature available on community groups and support systems

Additional information

Resuscitation

➲ Consider gastric lavage or activated charcoal if large quantity of substance taken and/or presentation is within 1 hour on ingestion
➲ IV access
➲ Inform ITU if patient is compromised on presentation

Toxbase

Toxbase is the UK National Poisons Information Service database (*see* www.toxbase.org).

SADPERSONS scale	Score
Sex (male)	1
Age (<19 and >45)	1
Depression or hopelessness	2
Previous attempts or psychiatric care	1
Excessive alcohol or drug use	1
Rational thinking loss (psychiatric or organic illness)	2
Separated, widowed or divorced	1
Organised or serious attempt	2
No social support	1
State future intent	2

➲ Score <6: may be safe for discharge (consider circumstances)
➲ Score 6–8: requires psychiatric review
➲ Score >8: candidate for hospital admission with psychiatric review

Specific poisons and antidotes

Poison	Antidote
Beta blockers	Glucagon, Actrapid
Cyanide	Sodium nitrate, sodium thiosulphate
Digoxin	Digibind (Digoxin antibody)
Ethylene glycol	Ethanol
Methanol	Ethanol
Opioids	Naloxone
Organophosphates	Atropine
Paracetamol	Acetylcysteine

Blood tests

⮞ Arterial blood gas as indicated

⮞ Venous: FBC, U&E, LFTs, glucose

⮞ Glucose level (capillary)

⮞ Paracetamol and salicylate levels at 4 hours post ingestion of substance:

   • for staggered overdoses, consult Toxbase

Alcohol intoxication[2,3]

1. Assess level of intoxication
2. Full physical examination and CAGE assessment
3. Bloods
4. Continuous reassessment and physiological monitoring
5. Referral or discharge

Admission:
- ➲ if patient remains intoxicated, admit for observation
- ➲ senior review to exclude another diagnosis

Discharge:
- ➲ prior to discharge patients should be ambulant, orientated and other coexisting medical problems excluded
- ➲ referral to local drug and alcohol team on discharge

Additional information

Assessing the level of intoxication

If reduced level of consciousness:
- ➲ ABCDE approach
- ➲ secure airway
- ➲ oxygen – ensure saturations 94%–98%
- ➲ blood glucose
- ➲ investigate other causes of unconsciousness (e.g. hypoglycaemia, intra-cranial bleed)
- ➲ senior review.

If violent:
- ➲ maintain safety (ensure security are present in department)
- ➲ blood glucose
- ➲ not to be discharged until all other causes have been investigated and excluded
- ➲ senior review prior to discharge.

CAGE

➲ **C** Have you ever felt you should *cut down* your drinking?

➲ **A** Have people *annoyed* you by criticising your drinking?

➲ **G** Have you ever felt *guilty* about your drinking?

➲ **E** Have you ever had an *eye-opener* drink first thing in the morning?

Blood tests

➲ Arterial blood gas if indicated

➲ Venous: FBC, U&E, LFTs, clotting, glucose

Alcohol withdrawal[2,3]

1. Identify those at risk and confirm diagnosis
2. Bloods
3. Commence reducing regimen of benzodiazepine as per local policy
4. Vitamin supplements should be prescribed in all cases of chronic alcohol
5. Continuous reassessment and physiological monitoring
6. Admission to ward for observation

Additional information

Key points in history and signs of withdrawal

History to include

- Substances used, duration and when last used
- Symptoms experienced and chronology
- Past interventions, treatment and outcomes
- Extent of any associated health and social problems
- Need for assisted alcohol withdrawal

Signs of withdrawal

- ↑HR, ↓BP, tremor, confusion, fits, hallucinations
- Occurs 24–72 hours after last drink

Classic triad of Wernicke

- Confusion, ataxia, nystagmus or ophthalmoplegia

Blood tests

- Venous: FBC, U&E, clotting, LFTs, glucose

Example of reducing regimen of benzodiazepine

- Chlordiazepoxide PO qds:
  - Day 1 – 30 mg qds
  - Day 2 – 30 mg tds
  - Day 3 – 20 mg tds
- Chlordiazepoxide 5 mg prescribed prn
- Dose may need to be altered depending on effect

Vitamin supplements

⮕ Use vitamin supplements to avoid Wernicke's encephalopathy as per local policy, e.g. Pabrinex (IV) or IM or PO agents available

⮕ If Wernicke's encephalopathy suspected, Pabrinex as two pairs tds for 3 days and review

Substance misuse

1. Assess reason for presentation
2. Full history and examination
3. Chronic cases are best managed in the community or primary care setting
4. Refer the patient on discharge to his or her GP and/or local drug or alcohol services
5. Provide any literature available on community groups and support systems

Additional information

History and examination

⮞ Full examination to exclude other pathology
⮞ Analgesia should not be withheld if patient is complaining of pain

When to consider discharge

⮞ Other medical conditions are excluded
⮞ If the patient is ambulant, orientated and safe discharge is appropriate

Panic or anxiety[4]

1. History and mental health assessment
2. Full physical examination to exclude any organic causes
3. Ascertain any precipitating factors or patterns to panic or anxiety
4. Talk through any symptoms such as palpitations and provide reassurance
5. Advise patient to seek advice from GP for longer-term management of symptoms

Additional information

Examination and investigations
⊃ Undertake the minimum investigations necessary to exclude acute physical problems

Also consider
⊃ Any co-morbid substance misuse
⊃ Any co-morbid medical condition
⊃ A history of mental health disorders
⊃ Past experience of, and response to, treatments

GP referral
⊃ Supply appropriate written information about panic attacks and why the patient is being referred to primary care
⊃ Offer appropriate written information about sources of support, including local and national voluntary and self-help groups

Acute psychosis[5]

1. History and mental health assessment
2. Full physical examination to exclude any organic causes
3. Early psychiatric referral and input
4. If cause for presentation is unknown, the treatment should be given cautiously under specialist advice
5. Maintain a safe and secure environment for the patient

Additional information

History

If the person has used substances, ask him or her about all of the following:
➜ particular substance(s) used
➜ quantity, frequency and pattern of use
➜ route of administration
➜ duration of current level of use.

Early psychiatric input

➜ Request background to past psychiatric history if known by psychiatric team

Possible first-line medication

➜ Olanzapine 10 mg PO

References

1. National Institute for Health and Clinical Excellence. *Self-Harm: NICE guideline 16*. London: NICE; 2004. www.nice.org.uk/CG16
2. National Institute for Health and Clinical Excellence. *Alcohol-Use Disorders: NICE guideline 100*. London: NICE; 2010. www.nice.org.uk/CG100
3. National Institute for Health and Clinical Excellence. *Alcohol Dependence and Harmful Alcohol Use: NICE guideline 115*. London: NICE; 2011. www.nice.org.uk/CG115
4. National Institute for Health and Clinical Excellence. *Anxiety: NICE guideline 113*. London: NICE; 2011. www.nice.org.uk/CG113
5. National Institute for Health and Clinical Excellence. *Psychosis with Coexisting Substance Misuse: NICE guideline 120*. London: NICE; 2011. www.nice.org.uk/CG120

Index

CPD with Radcliffe

You can now use a selection of our books to achieve CPD (Continuing Professional Development) points through directed reading.

We provide a free online form and downloadable certificate for your appraisal portfolio. Look for the CPD logo and register with us at: www.radcliffehealth.com/cpd

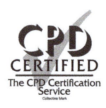